Miracle foods for kids

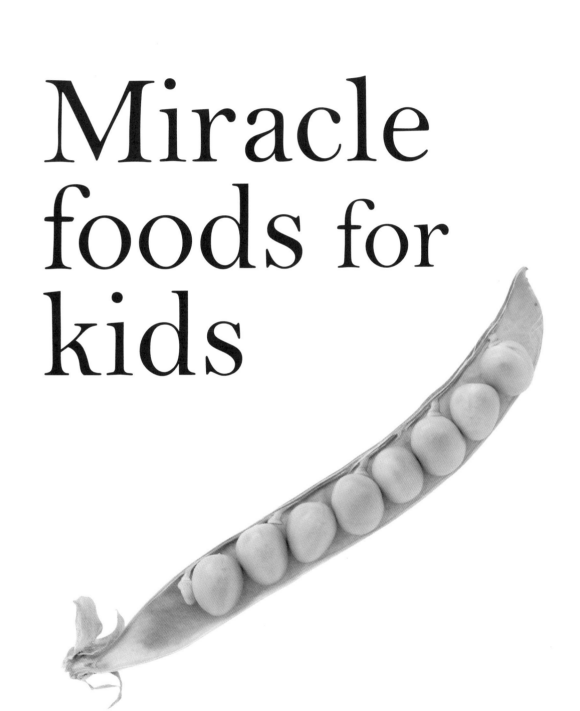

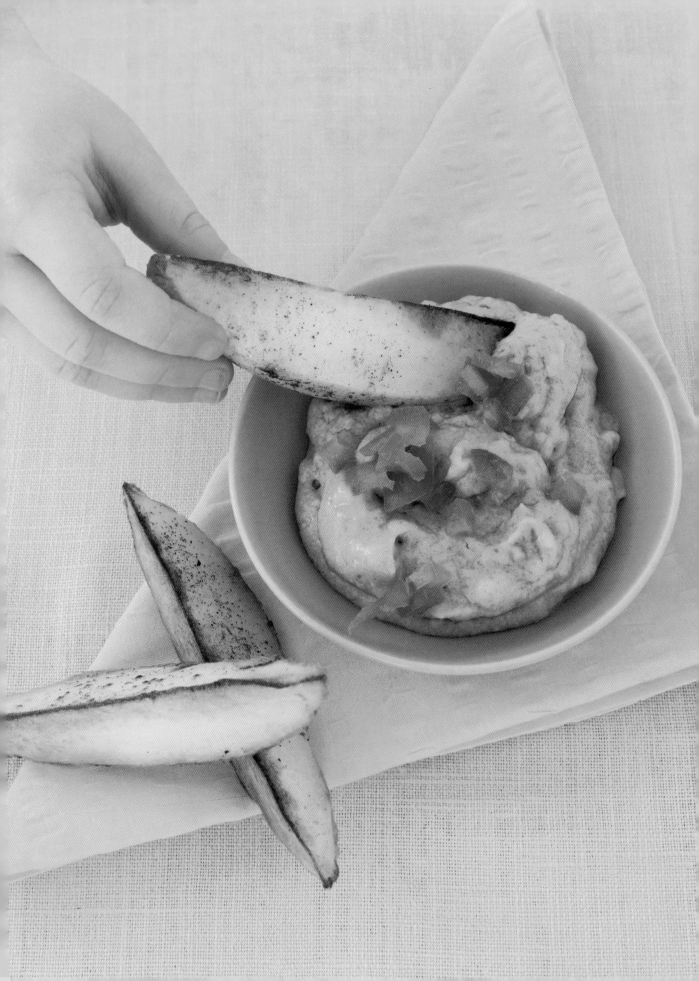

hamlyn

Miracle foods for kids

25 super-nutritious foods to keep your children in great health

Juliette Kellow

Recipes by
Sunil Vijayakar

First published in Great Britain in 2006 by
Hamlyn, a division of Octopus Publishing Group Ltd
2–4 Heron Quays, London E14 4JP

ISBN-13: 978-0-60061-455-5
ISBN-10: 0-600-61455-7

The moral right of the author has been asserted.

A CIP catalogue record for this book is available
from the British Library

Printed and bound in China

10 9 8 7 6 5 4 3 2 1

Notes

Miracle foods should not be considered a replacement
for professional medical treatment; a physician should
be consulted on all matters relating to health. While
the advice and information in this book is believed
to be accurate, neither the author or the publisher can
accept any legal responsibility for any injury or illness
sustained while following the advice in this book.

Both metric and imperial measurements have been given
in all recipes. Use one set of measurements only, and not
a mixture of both.

Ovens should be preheated to the specified temperature –
if using a fan-assisted oven, follow the manufacturer's
instructions for adjusting the time and the temperature.

The Department of Health advises that eggs should not
be consumed raw. This book contains dishes made with
raw or lightly cooked eggs. It is prudent for more
vulnerable people such as pregnant and nursing mothers,
invalids, the elderly, babies and young children to avoid
uncooked or lightly cooked dishes made with eggs.

This book includes dishes made with nuts and nut
derivatives. It is advisable for those with known allergic
reactions to nuts and nut derivatives and those who may
be potentially vulnerable to these allergies, such as
pregnant and nursing mothers, invalids, the elderly,
babies and children, to avoid dishes made with nuts
and nut oils.

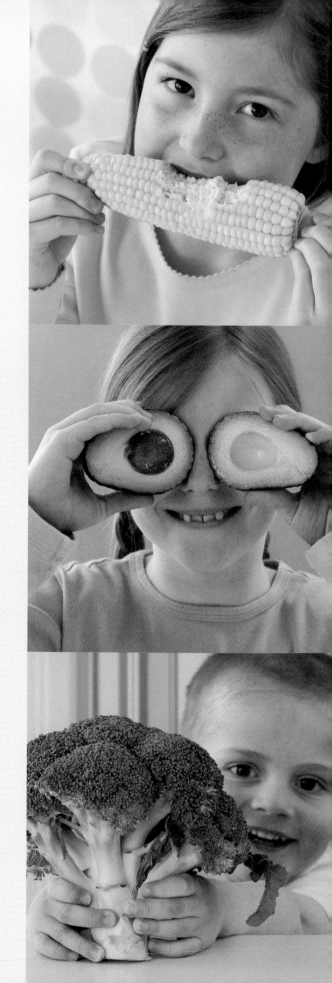

Contents

Miracle eating 6

Miracle foods 24

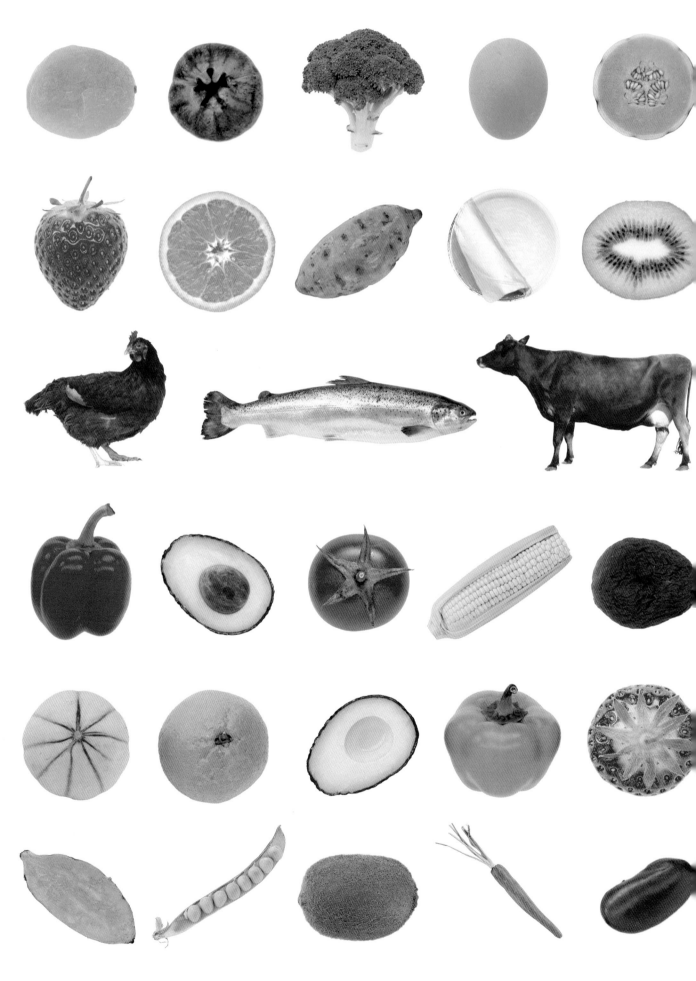

Part 1
Miracle eating

What are miracle foods?

As parents, we want the best for our children and that includes making sure they stay fit and healthy – not just when they are children and teenagers, but into adulthood. One of the best ways to achieve this is to provide them with healthy food in the early years and teach them the importance of eating a healthy, balanced diet as they get older, so they continue to make good choices throughout life.

Of course, it's well established that a balanced diet is essential for growth and development. But there is growing evidence that certain foods can make a significant difference to children's physical and mental health, both in the short- and long-term.

Making healthier choices

For example, most parents know a piece of fruit is a healthier choice than sweets or that kids should be eating more vegetables. But they probably don't know that oranges may prevent asthma, blueberries may boost memory or carrots fight infection. Needless to say, making the healthier option organic is even better; the availability of organic fruit and vegetables has increased dramatically over the past five years and most supermarkets sell a good range of organic produce.

This book highlights 25 of the most nutritious, health-promoting Miracle Foods you can encourage your child to eat and better still, they're foods you can buy at the supermarket with your weekly shop. While most help to protect against many health problems in later life such as heart disease, cancer, diabetes, osteoporosis, high blood pressure, arthritis and cataracts, they also have many more immediate benefits for children.

As well as promoting normal growth and development, some of these Miracle Foods help to prevent health problems frequently seen in children, such as obesity, constipation, anaemia and tooth decay. They can help cuts and bruises heal quickly or boost immunity so children are less likely to get coughs, colds or other infections that leave them needing time off school. They can even help to prevent or ease the symptoms of allergies such as asthma or eczema.

Brain-power boosters

But that's not all. Some Miracle Foods are great for kids who have behavioural problems or suffer with Attention Deficit Hyperactivity Disorder (ADHD). Many of the foods have a calming effect, so help to ease exam stress or the anxiety associated with going through puberty. Some will even help kids sleep better or help them to get more from their education by boosting memory and concentration and increasing brain power and IQ. Also importantly for teenagers, many of these foods can help them look good by encouraging spot-free skin, glossy hair and strong nails.

Some of these Miracle Foods are probably already part of your child's diet – but perhaps aren't being eaten regularly enough. Believe it or not, carrots, peas, sweetcorn, tomatoes, oranges, milk, yogurt, beef, chicken, rice and eggs are all Miracle Foods, with the result that many parents are probably well on the way to giving their children a nutritional boost at mealtimes.

In contrast, some Miracle Foods, like melon, strawberries, apricots, kiwifruit, peppers, broccoli, oats and cod may only make an occasional appearance on your child's plate – but you'll find there are plenty of reasons to serve them up more frequently. And other Miracle Foods may be competely new to your child or perhaps have only been tried once and instantly dismissed. But foods like avocado, sweet potatoes, kidney beans, blueberries, sunflower seeds and salmon have so many health-promoting nutrients it's a shame not to try them again, and again, until they become a regular part of your child's diet.

Free-radical buster

All our Miracle Foods provide a range of nutrients, but you'll see the buzz word 'antioxidants' repeated time and time again. Antioxidants are natural substances found in some foods that help to mop up potentially harmful molecules called free radicals. These free radicals are created naturally as a side-effect of metabolism but levels can increase dramatically when children and adults are exposed to health baddies such as cigarette smoke or pollution. This is bad news because free radicals can damage cells in the long term, causing heart disease, cancer, arthritis, cataracts and even asthma. That's why it's so important to get kids into the habit of eating plenty of antioxidant-rich foods – quite simply, the more antioxidants children have in their diet, the more potential they have to prevent health problems from developing, both now and in the future.

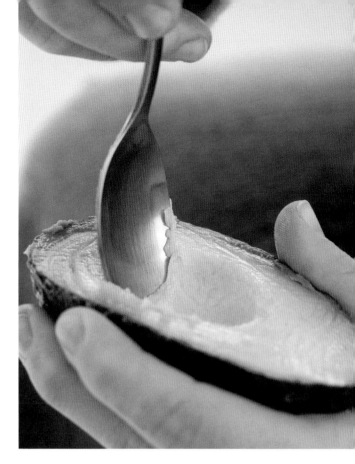

Encouraging a healthy diet

While eating more Miracle Foods is important, it's also essential that your child's overall diet is balanced and healthy – after all, encouraging children to eat a handful of blueberries or a few sunflower seeds is unlikely to do much good if most of the time they're still filling up on foods packed with saturated fats, sugar and salt, but few vitamins and minerals.

As the foundations for future good health and eating patterns are developed in the first few years of life, it's important to encourage good eating habits as soon as possible. Nevertheless, low-fat, high-fibre diets recommended for adults are unsuitable for most children under the age of five, as they may not get enough energy and nutrients for growth.

As young children only have small tummies they can't eat large amounts, so meals and snacks need to be packed with calories and nutrients. A diet containing good amounts of fat helps to ensure children get enough calories to grow properly, as well as providing essential fatty acids and the fat-soluble vitamins A and D. For this reason, children under the age of two shouldn't be given low-fat foods such as skimmed or semi-skimmed milk. But it's best for children to get fats from foods that contain other nutrients such as full-fat milk, meat and oily fish, rather than from foods that are high in fat but contain few vitamins and minerals, such as cakes, biscuits and chocolate.

Young children shouldn't be given too many fibre-rich foods either, as these may fill them up so much they can't eat enough to provide them with adequate calories and nutrients. Too much fibre can also cause tummy ache, diarrhoea or even constipation, if insufficient fluids are given, and may interfere with the absorption of minerals such as iron, calcium and zinc.

At least five-a-day

As children approach school age, they should gradually move towards a diet that is lower in fat and higher in fibre. And by the age of five, their diet should be low in fat, sugar and salt and high in fibre with five fruits and vegetables a day – just like adults.

Whatever their age, children can easily get a balanced diet by eating a variety of foods from four main food groups:

- Bread, other cereals and potatoes – these starchy foods, which also include pasta and rice, provide energy, fibre, vitamins and minerals.
- Fruit and vegetables – these provide fibre, vitamins and minerals and are a source of antioxidants.
- Milk and dairy foods – these provide calcium for healthy bones and teeth, protein for growth, plus vitamins and minerals.
- Meat, fish and alternatives – these foods, which include eggs and pulses, provide protein and vitamins and other minerals, especially iron. Pulses also contain fibre.

In contrast, foods from a fifth food group that includes fatty and sugary foods such as biscuits, cakes, fizzy drinks, chocolate, sweets, sugar, potato snacks and pastries, should be limited.

Do children need supplements?

In general, it's better for children and teenagers to get all the vitamins and minerals they need from a balanced diet, rather than supplements. Research shows that individual nutrients in the form of supplements are less likely to promote health compared with the combination of nutrients supplied in foods, and some supplements may even do more harm than good.

However, health experts believe children between the ages of six months and five years could benefit from taking drops containing vitamins A, C and D, particularly if they are not eating a varied diet. Vitamin D is also made in the body by the action of sunlight on skin. So if children are always inside, never expose their skin when they are outside or don't eat many foods rich in vitamin D (oily fish, eggs or fortified breakfast cereals), it's sensible to give them drops to boost intakes of this vitamin. Vitamin drops can be bought from child health clinics or pharmacies. Ask your health visitor or GP for more information.

Vitamin and mineral requirements for children and teenagers

Use this table to discover how Miracle Foods contribute to a balanced diet for children of different ages.

Nutrient	Daily vitamin and mineral requirements						
	1–3 years	4–6 years	7–10 years	11–14 years		15–18 years	
				Boys	Girls	Boys	Girls
VITAMINS							
Vitamin A (mcg)	400	500	500	600	600	700	600
Vitamin B1 (mg)	0.5	0.7	0.7	0.9	0.7	1.1	0.8
Vitamin B2 (mg)	0.6	0.8	1	1.2	1.1	1.3	1.1
Vitamin B3 (mg)	8	11	12	15	12	18	14
Vitamin B6 (mg)	0.7	0.9	1	1.2	1	1.5	1.2
Vitamin B12 (mcg)	0.5	0.8	1	1.2	1.2	1.5	1.5
Folate (mcg)	70	100	150	200	200	200	200
Vitamin C (mg)	30	30	30	35	35	40	40
Vitamin D (mcg)*	7	-	-	-	-	-	-
MINERALS							
Calcium (mg)	350	450	550	1,000	800	1,000	800
Phosphorus (mg)	270	350	450	775	625	775	625
Magnesium (mg)	85	120	200	280	280	300	300
Potassium (mg)	800	1,100	2,000	3,100	3,100	3,500	3,500
Iron (mg)	6.9	6.1	8.7	11.3	14.8	11.3	14.8
Zinc (mg)	5	6.5	7	9	9	9.5	7
Copper (mg)	0.4	0.6	0.7	0.8	1	0.8	1
Selenium (mcg)	15	20	30	45	45	70	60
Iodine (mcg)	70	100	110	130	130	140	140

*No values are set for children and teenagers after the age of three as sunlight is the main source of this vitamin.

Source: *Dietary Reference Values for Food Energy and Nutrients for the United Kingdom*, Department of Health.

How children's diets should vary from adults'

Our Miracle Foods include milk, yogurt, eggs, salmon, cod, sunflower seeds, many fruits and vegetables and several other high-fibre foods. These are all health heroes for children, but with little tummies in mind, it's important to follow a few guidelines.

Milk and dairy products

From the age of one, children can drink cows' milk, but give full-fat milk as it provides the extra calories and vitamins A and D that younger children need. From two years, semi-skimmed milk can be introduced, provided children are eating well, but wait until children are five before switching to skimmed milk. The same guidelines apply to yogurt – give full-fat yogurt to those under two, then consider introducing lower-fat yogurts.

High-fibre foods

Don't give children under two lots of filling, fibre-rich foods such as wholemeal pasta and brown rice. But gradually increase the amount of high-fibre foods offered after this time, so that by the age of five, children are eating plenty of fibre-rich foods.

Fruits and vegetables

Most fruits and vegetables make good weaning foods and should be encouraged throughout childhood. By five, children should be eating at least five portions every day.

Eggs

Raw eggs and foods containing raw or partially cooked eggs shouldn't be given to under-fives because of the risk of salmonella food poisoning. There's no need for young children to avoid eggs; just make sure they are cooked until both the white and yolk are solid. It is a good idea to buy free-range eggs, preferably organic.

Nuts and seeds

Children under the age of five shouldn't be given whole or chopped nuts and seeds because of the risk of choking. Instead, try crushing or flaking them.

Fish

Deep-sea fish such as shark, swordfish and marlin should be off-limits until children reach 16 years as these may contain mercury, which can affect the developing nervous system. With oily fish such as salmon, trout, sardines, mackerel, pilchards and fresh tuna, boys can have up to four portions a week, while girls should limit it to two portions a week (with a portion weighing 140 g/4½ oz). Girls should eat less because oily fish may contain pollutants that can build up in the body and be detrimental in later life to an unborn baby. It's also sensible to avoid giving uncooked shellfish to young children to reduce the risk of food poisoning.

Salt

While adults should have no more than 6 g of salt a day, children need even less as they have smaller bodies. Don't add salt to cooking or meals and check information on labels when you buy processed foods such as savoury snacks, ready-meals and sauces – even if they are aimed at children. Opt for those with the least sodium, since it is the sodium in salt that is linked to health problems such as high blood pressure. Processed meats like bacon, ham and sausages are also high in salt so limit these, too. The maximum amounts of salt children should have at different ages are as follows:

• 1–3 years: 2 g a day (0.8 g sodium)
• 4–6 years: 3 g a day (1.2 g sodium)
• 7–10 years: 5 g a day (2 g sodium)
• 11 years upwards: 6 g a day (2.5 g sodium)

Vitamins and minerals

Vitamins and minerals are only needed in tiny amounts but they are essential for good health. As the body can't make vitamins (except for D and K), they must be provided in the diet.

A child's age, gender, body size and activity levels affect their need for vitamins and minerals so recommended intakes often differ between boys and girls and different aged children. Older children usually need more of most vitamins and minerals than younger children because they are bigger. Similarly, boys over the age of 10 often need more of some vitamins and minerals than girls, with the exception of iron, where teenage girls need more to make up losses due to menstruation.

In the UK, recommended daily intakes for most vitamins and minerals are called Reference Nutrient Intakes (RNIs) — see the table on page 11. If your child usually meets the RNI, the risk of them being deficient in that nutrient is small. Recommended Daily Allowances (RDAs) and Guideline Daily Amounts (GDAs) found on some food labels are designed specifically for food labelling and are similar to, but not always the same as RNIs. However, these are based on nutritional needs for adults and shouldn't be applied to children.

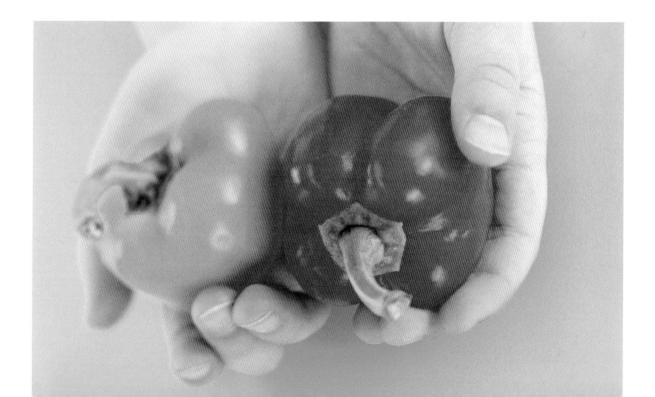

Nutrients children need

Most of our miracle foods are packed with a variety of vitamins and minerals. Check the table below to discover the role of these different nutrients in the body and their main food sources.

Nutrients and their sources

Nutrient	Why children need it	Food sources of nutrient	Miracle Food source
Vitamin A (Retinol and beta-carotene)	Important for growth, fighting infection, good vision and healthy skin. Beta-carotene (which the body uses to make vitamin A) is an antioxidant	Retinol is in full-fat dairy products: eggs, liver, margarine, Beta-carotene is in dark green and orange, red and yellow fruits and vegetables	Carrots, Eggs, Milk (full-fat), Peppers, Sweet potatoes
Vitamin B1	Needed for energy release, growth and a healthy nervous system	Wholegrain cereals, oats, brown rice, dairy products, yeast extract, pulses, nuts, seeds, pork and offal	Brown rice, Kidney beans, Oats, Peas, Sunflower seeds
Vitamin B2	Needed for energy release, growth and healthy eyes, skin, hair and nails	Dairy products, eggs, meat, offal, fortified breakfast cereals, almonds and yeast extract	Beef, Eggs, Milk, Yogurt
Vitamin B3	Releases energy from nutrients, controls blood sugar and keeps the skin, nervous and digestive systems healthy	Red meat, poultry, fish, eggs, nuts, potatoes, pasta, yeast extract, bread and breakfast cereals	Beef, Chicken, Cod, Eggs, Oats, Peas, Salmon, Sunflower seeds
Vitamin B6	Important for protein metabolism and making red blood cells and neurotransmitters	Fish, offal, red meat, yeast extract, soya beans, wholegrains, peanuts, walnuts, avocado and bananas	Avocado, Beef, Chicken, Cod, Peppers, Salmon
Vitamin B12	Needed for red blood cells, normal nerve function, growth and energy production	Meat, fish, chicken, eggs, milk, cheese, yogurt and breakfast cereals	Beef, Chicken, Cod, Eggs, Milk, Salmon, Yogurt
Folate	Needed to make red blood cells and protect against birth defects	Green vegetables, oranges, fortified breakfast cereals, yeast extract, nuts and pulses	Broccoli, Kidney beans, Oranges, Peas
Vitamin C	An antioxidant, important for healthy skin, bones, cartilage and teeth, wound-healing and aiding iron absorption	Blackcurrants, berries, green leafy vegetables, tomatoes, peppers, kiwifruit, citrus fruits and their juices	Blueberries, Broccoli, Kiwifruit, Melon, Oranges, Peas, Peppers, Strawberries, Sweet potatoes, Tomatoes

Nutrient	Why children need it	Food sources of nutrient	Miracle Food source
Vitamin D	Helps the body to absorb calcium so is important for strong bones and teeth	Sunshine. Food sources include oily fish, eggs, liver and fortified breakfast cereals and margarine	Salmon Eggs
Vitamin E	An antioxidant, helps heal wounds, prevents scarring and needed for healthy red blood cells and nerves	Vegetable oils, margarine, avocado, nuts, seeds, green leafy vegetables, eggs and wholegrains	Avocado, Blueberries Eggs, Oats, Peppers Salmon, Sunflower seeds, Sweet potatoes
Calcium	Essential for healthy bones and teeth, blood clotting and nerve impulse transmission	Milk, cheese, yogurt, pulses, nuts, seeds, fish eaten with the bones, dried fruit, green vegetables	Milk Sunflower seeds Yogurt
Phosphorus	Needed for strong bones, energy production and every chemical reaction in the body	Wholegrains, oats, yeast extract, nuts, seeds, dairy products, eggs, fish, offal, meat and pulses	Beef, Brown rice Chicken, Cod, Eggs Kidney beans, Milk Oats, Peas, Salmon Sunflower seeds Yogurt
Magnesium	Needed for healthy bones and proper nerve and muscle functioning	Nuts, seeds, wholegrains, green leafy vegetables	Brown rice, Oats Sunflower seeds Sweet potatoes
Potassium	Important for maintaining fluid balance and proper nerve and muscle function	Fresh and dried fruit, vegetables, nuts, seeds, avocado, fish	Apricots, Avocado Kidney beans Kiwi fruit, Melon Sunflower seeds
Iron	Essential for healthy blood	Red meat, oily fish, beans, lentils, eggs, green leafy vegetables, nuts, dried fruit, seeds and fortified breakfast cereals	Apricots Beef, Eggs Kidney beans Oats, Peas, Salmon Sunflower seeds
Zinc	Fights infection, boosts immunity and is needed for sexual development and reproduction	Meat, eggs, cheese, nuts and seeds	Beef, Chicken, Eggs, Oats Sunflower seeds
Copper	Important for iron and fat metabolism, a healthy heart and nervous system, healthy skin and hair, and immunity	Offal, nuts, seeds, shellfish	Apricots Avocado Brown rice, Oats Sunflower seeds
Selenium	An antioxidant, needed for the thyroid hormones	Nuts, seeds, offal, fish, pork, eggs, chicken	Sunflower seeds, Cod Salmon, Eggs, Chicken
Iodine	Needed for the thyroid hormones, which regulate metabolism and growth	Fish, peppers, dairy products, cereals, vegetables, fruit, eggs, meat	Cod, Milk Salmon Yogurt

Coping with poor eaters

Fussy eating, food fads and food refusal are common among young children as eating habits and preferences for foods start to develop. While distressing for parents, these are unlikely to have any long-term effects on children's health. As no single food is essential for growth and development, if children are still eating some foods from the four main food groups, it is unlikely they will be undernourished. In the meantime, follow these tips.

1 Monitor drinking habits

Children who fill up on fluids between meals won't feel hungry at mealtimes and may refuse to eat. To prevent this, don't allow too many drinks between meals, especially in the hour before a meal. Offer drinks at the end of a meal rather than during, so that hunger is satisfied with food rather than fluid. Stick with water or diluted fruit juice and don't use bottles after the first year – giving drinks in a cup or beaker will help to reduce the amount of fluids consumed.

2 Check snacking habits

Most toddlers have small appetites and snacks can help to provide the extra calories and nutrients needed for growth. But if children end up snacking too much they won't be hungry enough to eat at mealtimes. Offering fruit or vegetable sticks between meals rather than toast or cake means they'll feel hungrier at mealtimes.

3 Take the meal away

If children refuse to eat, take the meal away and don't offer anything else until the next mealtime. In particular, avoid giving sweets, cakes, biscuits and savoury snacks between meals. Toddlers may eat less than normal for a few days and be more troublesome, but healthy children will rarely starve themselves. Get the rest of the family on your side too – you don't want them undoing all your good work!

4 Stay calm

Children quickly learn they can disrupt mealtimes by refusing to eat or to try new foods. It's important to avoid constantly focusing on them, so avoid making a fuss or arguing with your child or other family members about food. And never force-feed.

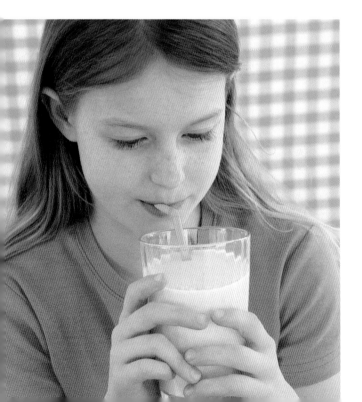

5 Keep offering new foods

Research shows the more frequently different foods are offered to children, the more likely they are to eat a varied diet later on, so don't be put off if your child refuses a new food the first time you offer it. Simply take it away and try it again in a few weeks' time, perhaps in a different form. You may need to offer new foods many times before a child starts to accept them, so don't give up.

6 Build on favourite foods

This is particularly important for children who will only eat a limited range of foods. For example, if your child loves milk, add a little banana to make a milkshake, make custard and serve with stewed apple, or make a cheese sauce and serve with vegetables.

7 Don't punish, but praise

Children rarely respond to punishment, but love to be praised. Give plenty of encouragement when children eat well. Set up a reward chart where they get a star for trying a new food.

8 Make mealtimes an occasion

Get children involved in mealtimes by letting them help, for example, by setting the table or helping to prepare food. Make the table look attractive – for younger children, use coloured tablecloths, plates and beakers. Letting children serve themselves may also encourage them to try new foods. Young children love to copy parents and older siblings, so if families eat together there's a greater chance younger children will join in.

9 Get the environment right

Children are easily distracted, so keep them focused on their food by making sure that toys, television and other distractions are out of sight at mealtimes.

10 Provide the right food

Make sure children can manage the food offered by cutting it into bite-sized pieces and have the correct-sized utensils. Hungry children who are unable to get food from the plate to their mouth will get frustrated and irritated.

How to get older children eating a more varied, healthier diet

- Buy lower-fat, lower-salt versions of favourites such as sausages, burgers and oven chips, then grill or oven bake these rather than frying – they'll never notice. The same goes for savoury snacks and biscuits!
- Sneak vegetables into dishes: add finely chopped red pepper to tomato sauces; grated carrot to Bolognese; and mashed cauliflower or leek to mashed potato.
- Serve big portions of vegetables that they like.
- Add beans, barley or lentils to soups and stews.
- Mix grated carrot and Red Leicester or Cheddar-type cheese and use to fill sandwiches or baked potatoes – the colours blend well so they won't notice the carrot.
- If you can't get your kids to give up sugary cereals, mix these with non-sugar varieties.
- For sandwiches, use spread on just one slice of bread or use reduced-fat mayonnaise in place of spread altogether.
- Use wholemeal pasta in pasta bakes – when mixed with sauce it is difficult to tell it's not white.
- For children who are resistant to brown rice or wholemeal pasta, cook half of each and then mix together.
- Get them to eat fruit by making smoothies or freeze pure orange juice in the shape of lollies.

Children's meal plans

Boys have higher calorie requirements than girls at all ages because they are generally bigger. After the age of ten, requirements for vitamins and minerals also differ, with boys having slightly higher requirements. The meal plans here are designed to meet the daily requirements for most children.

One to three years

- Let your child's appetite guide you on portion sizes for meals and snacks.
- Encourage healthy snacks such as fresh or dried fruit, yogurt or toast rather than biscuits, potato crisps and chocolate.
- Don't use low-fat or reduced-fat products for children under the age of two.
- Don't give too many high-fibre foods such as wholemeal bread or brown rice, especially for children under the age of two.
- The best drinks are milk and water. However, children like fruit juices, which are a good source of vitamin C and can count as one serving of the recommended five fruit and vegetables a day. But when juice is removed from the whole fruit, this releases natural sugars that can damage teeth. So to keep teeth healthy, only offer fruit juice at mealtimes and always put it in a cup rather than a bottle so that teeth aren't constantly in contact with the fluid.
- Offer a wide variety of foods and don't be put off if children initially refuse something. Keep trying.

Breakfast
Boiled egg with white toast and sunflower margarine; a banana

Snack
Raisins

Lunch
Pasta with minced beef, peas and homemade tomato sauce; seedless grapes

Snack
Mini pot of full-fat fruit yogurt

Dinner
Bread roll filled with full-fat soft cheese and tomato; orange segments

Drinks throughout the day
Around 600 ml (1 pint) milk; water; small cup unsweetened fruit juice diluted with water and given with a meal

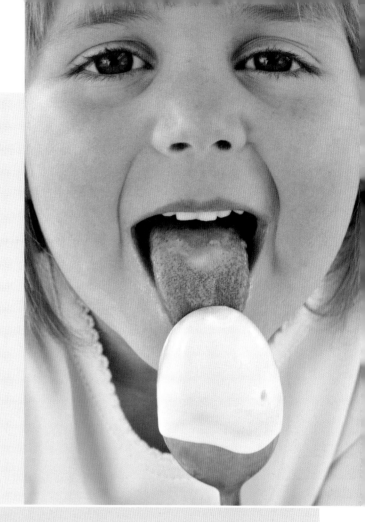

Four to six years

- Let your child's appetite and weight guide you on portion sizes for meals and snacks.
- Continue to encourage healthy snacks such as fresh or dried fruit, yogurt or toast rather than biscuits, potato crisps and chocolate.
- Gradually introduce more high-fibre foods such as wholemeal bread, wholemeal pasta, wholegrain cereals and brown rice. By the age of five, most children should be eating a diet that is higher in fibre. Make sure your child drinks enough fluids, too.
- The best drinks for children continue to be milk and water.
- If your child is eating well and growing, give semi-skimmed milk, but don't offer skimmed milk until after the age of five.
- Continue to increase the variety of foods offered to your child.

Breakfast
Wheat biscuit cereal with milk and strawberries

Snack
Banana

Lunch
School meal: Baked potato with butter, baked beans and salad; a pot of fruit yogurt
Packed lunch: Sandwich made with wholemeal bread filled with tuna and sweetcorn (both canned in water) and a little reduced-fat mayonnaise; cucumber sticks; slice of malt loaf and a pot of fruit yogurt

Snack
Wholemeal toast with peanut butter

Dinner
Homemade cottage pie (don't add salt) with broccoli and carrots;
stewed apple and custard made with semi-skimmed milk

Drinks throughout the day
Around 300 ml (½ pint) milk; water; one glass of unsweetened fruit juice diluted with water and drunk with a meal

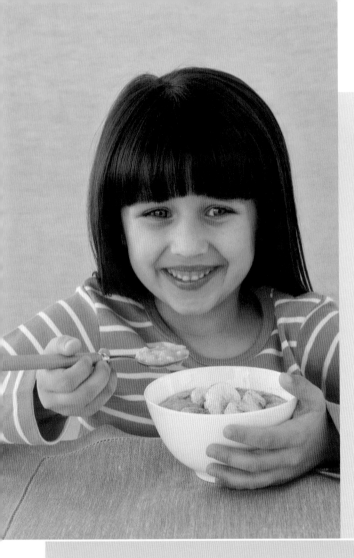

Seven to ten years

- Let your child's appetite and weight guide you on portion sizes for meals and snacks.
- By now your child should be eating a diet in line with healthy-eating guidelines for adults. Meals and snacks should be reasonably low in fat and high in fibre.
- Milk and water remain the best drinks. If your child won't drink milk, try blending it with favourite fruits to make a milkshake.
- Make sure children are eating five servings of fruit and vegetables every day – aim for a variety of colours to provide a good mix of nutrients.
- Talk to your children about the benefits eating well will have, such as helping them do better in lessons and at sports.

Breakfast
Porridge made with semi-skimmed milk and dried apricots; a glass of unsweetened orange juice

Snack
Small bag of mixed nuts; an apple

Lunch
School meal: Cheese and tomato pizza with salad; a bowl of fruit salad
Packed lunch: Wholemeal pitta bread filled with egg and tomato; pot of fruit fromage frais and a pear

Snack
Wholemeal toast with mashed banana

Dinner
Lamb and pepper kebabs with brown rice, salad and a yogurt and cucumber dip; wholemeal fruit crumble and custard made with semi-skimmed milk

Drinks throughout the day
Around 300 ml (½ pint) milk; water

Eleven to fourteen years

- Your teenager's appetite and weight should continue to be the main guide for portion sizes of meals and snacks.
- By now your teenager will probably be making more decisions about the food he or she wants to eat, especially outside of the home. Remember, children learn by example so make sure the whole family eats a healthy diet.
- Milk and water remain the best drinks.
- Provide children with healthy snacks in their school bag such as fruit, seeds or dried fruit.

Breakfast

Scrambled eggs on wholemeal toast with low-fat spread; a glass of unsweetened orange juice

Snack

A banana

Lunch

School meal: Fish cake, baked potato and peas; an apple

Packed lunch: Wholemeal bagel with low-fat soft cheese and tomato; an apple, pot of low-fat fruit yogurt and a handful of sunflower seeds

Snack

Hummus with carrot sticks

Dinner

Homemade spaghetti Bolognese with wholemeal pasta (don't add salt to either) and salad; fruit salad

Drinks throughout the day

450 ml (¾ pint) milk for girls and 600 ml (1 pint) milk for boys; water

Vegetarian diets for children

As with any diet, vegetarian diets shouldn't contain too many fatty, sugary or salty foods. They should also be balanced and include all the nutrients needed for good health. Meat, chicken and fish are important sources of protein, so vegetarian diets which omit these foods need to include alternative sources such as milk, cheese, yogurt, eggs, beans and lentils.

Meat is also packed with iron, so vegetarian diets should provide other iron-rich foods such as wholegrain cereals, eggs, green leafy vegetables, pulses, dried fruit, nuts and seeds, especially for teenage girls who have higher requirements for iron than boys. Vitamin C helps the body to absorb iron from plant foods, so foods rich in these two nutrients should be eaten together, for example, a glass of fruit juice with cereal. Tea should also be avoided at mealtimes as it contains tannins, which hinder iron absorption.

Fifteen to eighteen years

- Once again, your teenager's appetite and weight should remain the guide for portion sizes at meals and snacks.

- Milk and water remain the best drinks.
- Explain how eating well can help teenagers to look good.

Breakfast

Bran flake-type cereal with skimmed or semi-skimmed milk and raisins; wholemeal toast with peanut butter

Snack

A banana

Lunch

School lunch: Vegetable soup with a wholemeal cheese and tomato roll; fresh fruit salad

Packed lunch: Pasta salad made from wholemeal pasta, cherry tomatoes, chicken, favourite vegetables and a little reduced-fat mayonnaise; pot of low-fat fromage frais and seedless grapes

Snack

Fresh popcorn made without salt or sugar

Dinner

Grilled salmon and potatoes wedges brushed with olive oil, green beans and carrots; meringue nest filled with strawberries, blueberries and raspberries and a scoop of ice cream

Drinks throughout the day

450 ml (¾ pint) milk for girls and 600 ml (1 pint) milk for boys; water

School lunch vs packed lunch

School meals have received a lot of negative attention in recent years, with the result that many parents have opted to provide packed lunches for their children in order to guarantee that what their children consume is nutritious and healthy.

If your child has a school lunch, talk to him or her about the choices; try to encourage your child to vary the meals and opt for healthier options, such as pizza and salad, baked potatoes with baked beans or chilli with rice, rather than burgers, hot dogs, chicken nuggets and French fries.

If you choose to give your child a packed lunch, keep it as varied and interesting as possible – and make sure you pack in plenty of nutrients. Here's how to pack a nutritious lunch.

- Use wholegrain or wholemeal bread, rolls and pitta bread. For variety, try wraps, bagels, and raisin or sun-dried tomato bread.
- Cut fat by using less butter, spread or mayonnaise in sandwiches and rolls; choose low-fat fillings such as lean ham, turkey, chicken, tuna in water, eggs, cottage cheese, Edam or banana.
- Stop kids getting bored with sandwiches by switching them for pasta or rice salad,

How to get your kids to eat more fruit and vegetables

Many children refuse to eat fruit and vegetables as a way of asserting their new-found independence. However, fruit and vegetables provide many important vitamins and minerals. Children over the age of five should have at least five servings each day. Here are some ways to get your kids eating more:

Vegetables

- Offer vegetables your child may never have tried before such as pak choi, mangetout, artichokes, aubergine, bean sprouts, celeriac, fennel, endive and Chinese leaf.
- Cook vegetables in different ways. There's a world of difference between over-boiled soggy cabbage and lightly stir-fried cabbage. Try roasting parsnips, carrots, peppers, courgettes or cherry tomatoes.
- Add loads of vegetables to meat dishes such as casseroles, stews, spaghetti Bolognese, cottage pie or curries. For children who are adamant they won't eat vegetables, grate or cut these into small pieces so they're not easily identifiable.
- Add vegetables to favourite foods such as pizza, quiche, omelettes and sandwiches.
- Mix vegetables together – mashing parsnip with potato or carrots with swede.
- Offer raw vegetables such as pieces of carrot, celery, cucumber, pepper, tomato, mushroom and cauliflower with a favourite dip.

Fruit

- Offer fruits your child may never have tried before such as blueberries, figs, guava, kumquats, mango, passion fruit, pomegranates and star fruit.
- Purée fresh or canned fruit in juice and swirl into natural yogurt or serve with ice cream.
- Make fruit smoothies or milkshakes by blending with milk and yogurt.
- Add fresh or canned fruit in juice to jelly or mousse or serve with custard.
- Offer fruity puddings such as baked apple, fruit crumble, fruit salad, fruit flan or meringue nests filled with fruit.
- Offer a small glass of unsweetened fruit juice every day – try mixing it with still or sparkling water.
- Chop fresh fruit into bite-sized pieces for young children to make it easier to eat.
- Offer mini boxes of dried fruit such as raisins or small packs of apricots or mixed fruit – kids will eat them like sweets.

homemade pizza or wholegrain crackers with toppings.
- In the winter, pack a flask of homemade vegetable or tomato soup.
- Add two portions of fruit but don't just stick to apples and pears – include grapes, fruit salad, melon, a handful of blueberries or strawberries, small boxes of raisins or cans of fruit in their own juice.
- Include cherry tomatoes, carrot and pepper sticks and add salad to sandwiches.
- Replace cakes, biscuits and chocolate with scones, fruit bread or low-sugar cereal bars (check the labels)

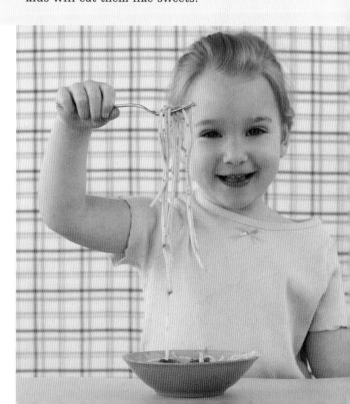

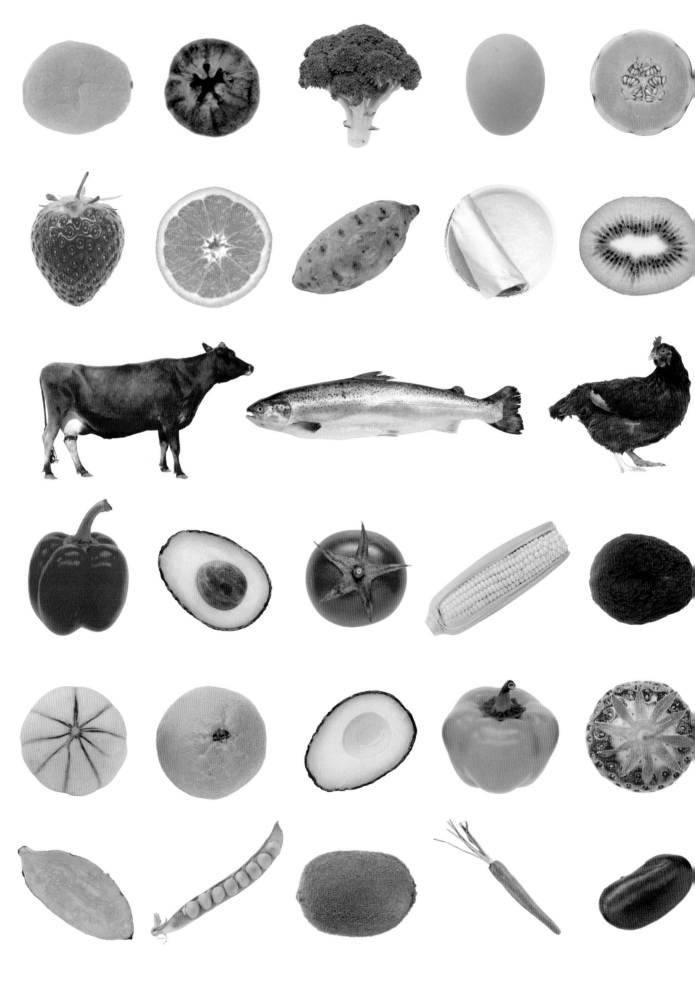

Part 2
Miracle foods

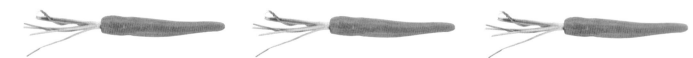

Carrots

What's in them?
Boiled carrots

Nutrients	100 g (3½ oz)	40 g (1 tbsp)
Calories	24 kcal	10 kcal
Protein	0.6 g	0.2 g
Fat	0.4 g	0.2 g
Carb	4.9 g	2 g
Fibre	2.5 g	1 g
Vitamin A	1,260 mcg	504 mcg

Benefits
- Help eyesight
- Boost immunity
- Aid healthy lungs

Carrots don't just help children see in the dark, they may also ease asthma, boost immunity and protect against passive smoking.

Keen on carotene

Carrots might be a favourite vegetable for children because of their bright colour and sweet taste, but the abundance of beta-carotene also makes them a health winner. As well as being an antioxidant, beta-carotene is converted into vitamin A in the body and this vitamin is essential for growth. Carrots are an especially important food for children as many have low intakes of vitamin A. The UK's latest National Diet and Nutrition Survey of Young People revealed that up to 13 per cent of boys and 20 per cent of girls have vitamin A intakes below the minimum amount needed for good health, with teenagers suffering the most.

Right for sight

Carrots really do help children see in the dark. Vitamin A is transformed into the purple pigment rhodopsin in the retina, which is essential for vision in dim light. According to the World Health Organization around 1.4 million children in the world are blind mainly due to vitamin A deficiency, highlighting how important this nutrient is for sight.

Fight infections

Getting kids to eat carrots may boost immunity. Vitamin A keeps healthy the skin and cells that line the airways, digestive tract and urinary tract – these form the body's first line of defence against infection. Even mild vitamin A deficiencies in children are linked to higher incidences of respiratory disease and diarrhoea.

Breathe easy

Carrots may prevent asthma in children, especially in kids regularly surrounded by smokers. A study of 4–16 year-olds

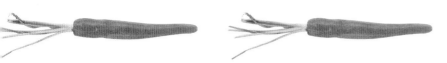
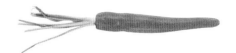

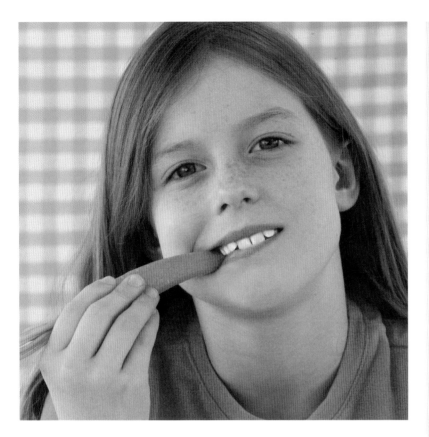

found good intakes of beta-carotene reduced asthma by 10 per cent in those in smoke-free environments, and by 40 per cent in those exposed to passive smoke. Other research shows that a carcinogen in cigarette smoke induces vitamin A deficiency, making it even more important for children to get good intakes of this nutrient if they are exposed to second-hand smoke. It's important children get this nutrient from food rather than supplements. Research shows that beta-carotene supplements may be harmful.

Give carrots the crunch

Don't worry if your kids will only eat mashed carrot – it's a nutritional bonus as more beta-carotene is absorbed from cooked, puréed carrots than from raw ones. Add butter to boiled carrots or roast them in olive oil, too, as fat helps the body to absorb beta-carotene.

Won't eat...
Boiled carrots

Might eat...
Raw carrot sticks with a dip

Will eat...
Carrot soup with cheesy toast

Three ways
to get your kids to eat more carrots

1 Fill baked potatoes or sandwiches with grated carrot and Red Leicester cheese.

2 Purée, mash or roast carrots with other root vegetables such as potatoes, parsnips or swede.

3 Add grated carrots to salad, stews or soups.

Why not try...
Carrot spice cake
(see page 28)
Nutritional facts per slice
283 kcal, 15.3 g fat (of which 2.3 g saturates), 20.7 g sugars, 0.3 g salt

Carrot and red cabbage slaw in pitta pockets
(see page 28)
Nutritional facts per pocket
120 kcal, 2.1 g fat (of which 0.1 g saturates), 5.8 g sugars, 0.6 g salt

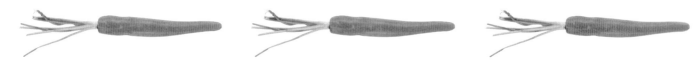

Carrot spice cake

● Preparation time **20 mins** ● Cooking time **45–50 mins** ● Makes **12 slices**

225 g (7½ oz) **self-raising flour, sifted**
2 tsp **ground cinnamon**
1 tsp **ground ginger**
½ tsp **allspice**
225 g (7½ oz) **light muscovado sugar**
225 g (7½ oz) **carrots, coarsely grated**
4 **large eggs, lightly beaten**
150 ml (¼ pint) **olive or sunflower oil**

1 Grease and base-line a 20 cm (8 inch) springform cake tin. Put the flour, spices and sugar in a bowl and mix together. Add the carrots and mix to combine.

2 Whisk the eggs with the oil and add to the flour mixture. Mix well with a spoon.

3 Pour the mixture into the prepared cake tin and level the surface. Bake in a preheated oven, 180°C (350°C), Gas Mark 4, for 45–50 minutes or until cooked through and golden. Remove from the oven and allow to stand for 10–15 minutes before turning out on to a wire rack. Allow to cool before serving.

Carrot and red cabbage slaw in pitta pockets

● Preparation time **15 mins, plus standing** ● Makes **8**

Slaw
200 g (7 oz) **carrots, coarsely grated**
50 g (2 oz) **finely shredded red cabbage**
1 tbsp **raisins or sultanas**
2 tbsp **lemon juice**
To serve
4 **wholemeal pitta breads**
100 g (3½ oz) **hummus**

1 Make the slaw. Mix together all the ingredients in a bowl and leave to stand at room temperature for 12–15 minutes.

2 Lightly toast the pitta breads and carefully split them open. Spread some hummus inside each and then stuff them with the carrot slaw. Cut each pitta pocket in half and serve immediately.

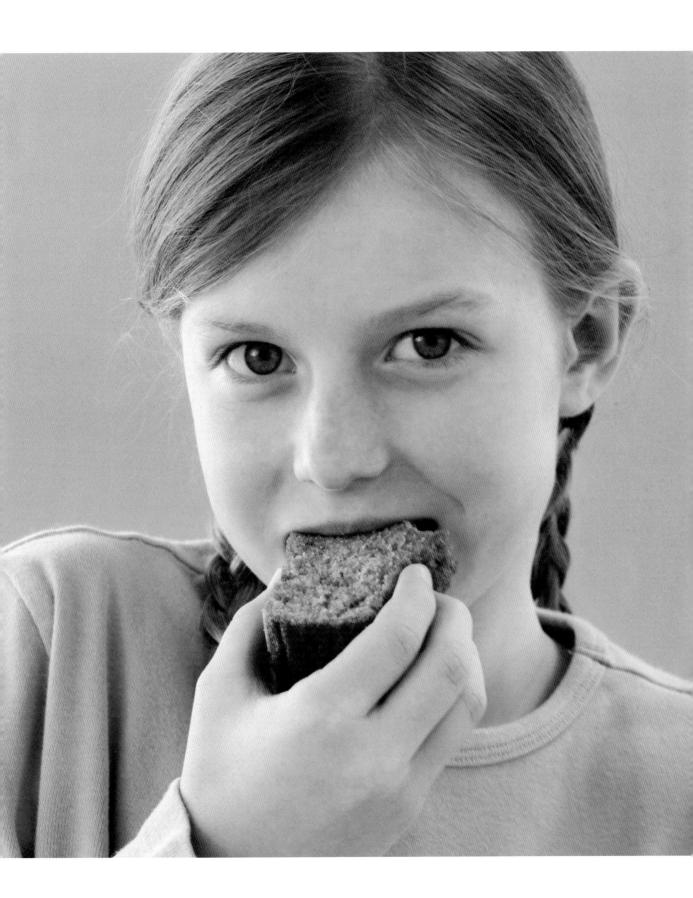

Broccoli

With its important vitamins and numerous health benefits, broccoli is one vegetable that should be on every parent's shopping list.

What's in it?
Steamed broccoli

Nutrients	100 g (3½ oz)	Per floret (45 g)
Calories	24 kcal	11 kcal
Protein	3.1 g	1.4 g
Fat	0.8 g	0.4 g
Carb	1.1 g	0.5 g
Fibre	2.3 g	1 g
Folate	64 mcg	29 mcg
Vitamin C	44 mg	20 mg
Vitamin E	1.1 mg	0.5 mg

Benefits

- Prevents tummy problems
- Protects eyes and skin from sunlight
- Helps to prevent cancer and heart disease

Nutritional powerhouse

It tastes great with cheese sauce and is the perfect accompaniment to roast dinners, but broccoli is also a nutritional powerhouse, containing good amounts of folate and vitamins C, E and K, smaller amounts of beta-carotene and potassium, and several health-promoting plant chemicals. Good news then that 13 per cent of children aged 4–16 list broccoli as their favourite vegetable according to a survey by The Stroke Association.

Prevent tummy troubles

Getting kids to eat broccoli may help to kill *Helicobacter pylori*, a bacteria linked with frequent tummy aches in children; it is also thought to be the major cause of chronic gastritis and duodenal ulcers in childhood. The magic bacteria-killing ingredient is a naturally occurring plant chemical called sulphoraphane. While antibiotics remain the main treatment for *H. pylori*, filling kids' plates with broccoli won't do any harm.

The coolest shades

Eating broccoli may help protect children's eyes from the harmful effects of sunlight. Broccoli contains two carotenoids – lutein and zeaxanthin – found in large amounts in the macula, a small area of the retina in the eye. As well as giving broccoli its green colour, these plant chemicals act as 'natural' sunglasses and filter out harmful light, stopping it from reaching and damaging the macula. They also mop up excess free radicals triggered by UV light, helping to prevent eye diseases such as cataracts. But that's not all. Broccoli contains two other eye-healthy nutrients: vitamin C (see Oranges), which may also prevent cataracts in later life; and beta-carotene, which the body uses to make vision vitamin, A (see Carrots).

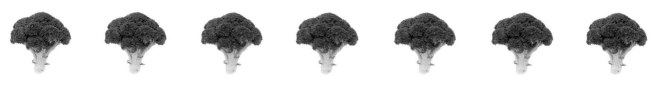

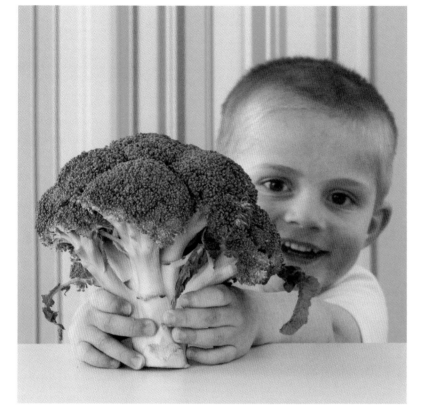

Great for growth

Broccoli is packed with the B vitamin folate, needed for cell reproduction, making red blood cells and preventing birth defects such as spina bifida. Broccoli is a particularly important source of this nutrient for kids as other folate-rich foods such as sprouts, spinach and cabbage are often unpopular.

Stops bleeding

Broccoli is a great choice for accident-prone kids because it is one of the few good food sources of vitamin K, a nutrient that promotes blood clotting to stop bleeding. Vitamin K is also made in the body by bacteria that live in the gut. So eating more broccoli may be important for children taking antibiotics as these can destroy the bacteria responsible for making this vitamin.

Looking forward

Brocoli may help to prevent age-related eye problems, peptic ulcers, cancer and heart disease in adults.

Won't eat...
Broccoli as a vegetable

Might eat...
Broccoli in a stir-fry

Will eat...
Broccoli and pasta covered with cheese sauce

Three ways
to get your kids to eat more broccoli

1 Add small broccoli florets to salads or use to top pizzas.

2 Serve raw florets with your child's favourite dip for a tasty snack.

3 Make broccoli soup and serve with wholegrain toast for a weekend lunch.

Why not try...

Broccoli and roasted red pepper pizzettas (see page 32)
Nutritional facts per pizza
258 kcal, 14.6 g fat (of which 4.3 g saturates), 3.4 g sugars, 0.5 g salt

Broccoli tagliatelle
(see page 32)
Nutritional facts per portion
252 kcal, 7.2 g fat (of which 1.1 g saturates), 3.9 g sugars, 0 g salt

Broccoli and roasted red pepper pizzettas

● Preparation time **30 mins, plus proving** ● Cooking time **about 35 mins** ● Makes **8**

Topping

1 **red pepper, halved lengthways**

300 g (10 oz) **broccoli, broken into small florets**

1 tbsp **olive oil**

2 **garlic cloves, crushed**

400 g (13 oz) **can chopped tomatoes**

2 tsp **dried oregano**

100 g (3½ oz) **Cheddar cheese, grated**

Pizzetta dough

50 g (2 oz) **wholemeal self-raising flour**

175 g (6 oz) **self-raising flour**

2 tsp **dried mixed herbs**

6 tbsp **olive oil**

150 ml (¼ pint) **water**

1 Prepare the topping. Place the pepper, cut side down, on a foil-lined grill pan. Grill until the skin is charred and blistered. Place in a plastic bag for 5–10 minutes then peel off the skin and discard the seeds. Roughly chop the flesh and set aside.

2 Blanch the broccoli florets in a pan of boiling water for 2–3 minutes, drain and set aside. Heat the olive oil in a nonstick frying pan. Add the garlic, fry for a minute, add the tomatoes and oregano and cook, stirring, for 10–12 minutes until thickened.

3 Make the dough. Mix together the flours, mixed herbs and 3 tablespoons of the oil. Add the water and mix to make a soft dough. Turn out the dough onto a lightly floured surface and knead for 5–6 minutes until smooth. Form into a ball, wrap in clingfilm and chill for 20–30 minutes.

4 Divide the dough into 8 and roll each piece into a circle about 6 cm (2½ inches) across. Heat half the remaining oil in a large, nonstick frying pan and arrange 4 of the pizzetta bases in the pan. Cook for 2–3 minutes on each side, remove and keep warm while you cook the remaining bases in the remaining oil.

5 Spread the tomato mixture over the bases and top each one with red pepper and broccoli florets. Sprinkle over the cheese and place under a preheated grill for 1–2 minutes.

Broccoli tagliatelle

● Preparation time **15 mins** ● Cooking time **14–19 mins** ● Serves **4**

200 g (7 oz) **tagliatelle**

300 g (10 oz) **broccoli, cut into small florets**

2 tbsp **olive oil**

1 **garlic clove, finely chopped**

10 **cherry tomatoes, halved**

pepper

1 Cook the tagliatelle according to the instructions on the packet. Drain and keep warm. Steam the broccoli for 2–3 minutes, drain and keep warm.

2 Heat the oil in a large, nonstick frying pan. Add the garlic and drained broccoli, stir-fry for 1–2 minutes and add the drained pasta and cherry tomatoes. Toss to mix well and cook, stirring, for 1–2 minutes. Season to taste, remove from the heat and serve immediately.

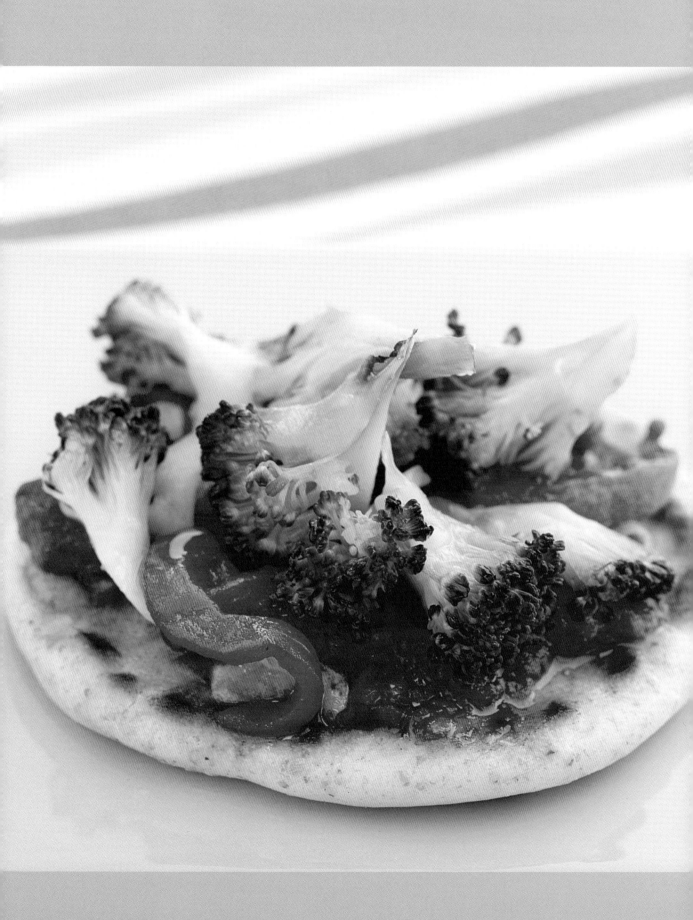

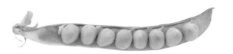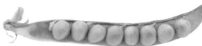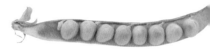

Peas

What's in them?
Frozen peas (boiled)

Nutrients	100 g (3½ oz)	Per tbsp (30 g)
Calories	69 kcal	21 kcal
Protein	6 g	1.8 g
Fat	0.9 g	0.3 g
Carb	9.7 g	2.9 g
Fibre	5.1 g	1.5 g
Vitamin B1	0.3 mg	0.1 mg
Vitamin B3	1.7 mg	0.5 mg
Folate	33 mcg	10 mcg
Vitamin C	12 mg	4 mg
Phosphorus	99 mg	30 mg
Iron	1.6 mg	0.5 mg

Benefits
- **Protein source for vegetarians**
- **May help ease diarrhoea**
- **Fight depression**
- **Boost concentration**
- **Prevent obesity, diabetes and heart disease**

Feel guilty because peas are the only vegetable your kids will eat? There's no need because peas are packed with nutrients to keep kids fighting fit.

Ap-pea-ling

Peas are the perfect accompaniment to fish fingers and chips, but their nutrient content makes them even more appealing. Peas are packed with several B vitamins, vitamin C and the minerals iron, phosphorus and manganese. They are also a good source of soluble fibre, the type that keeps blood-sugar levels steady, therefore helping to boost concentration, lower blood cholesterol and prevent hunger. This means they can have a role in protecting against obesity, diabetes and high-blood cholesterol (see Oats).

Peas for protein

Kids might think peas are a vegetable, but they are actually a legume, belonging to the same family as lentils and beans. This means that peas contain more protein than other vegetables, making them a good choice for vegetarian children. However, some of the essential amino acids (protein building-blocks) in peas are present only in very small amounts. But combine them with eggs, milk or cheese – which contain all of the essential amino acids – and the deficiency is supplemented. Adding peas to omelettes, quiches, cheese-topped pizzas or macaroni cheese is an excellent way to enhance the protein quality of peas for vegetarian children.

Dealing with diarrhoea

Thanks to their soluble fibre content, peas may help to ease diarrhoea. Soluble fibre dissolves in water to form a viscous mixture that binds the stools together and slows the passage of food through the digestive tract. But getting children to eat peas when they are unwell may not be easy – so try mixing them with mashed potato or pasta and tomato sauce.

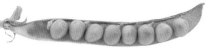 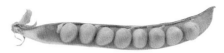 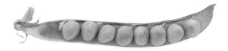

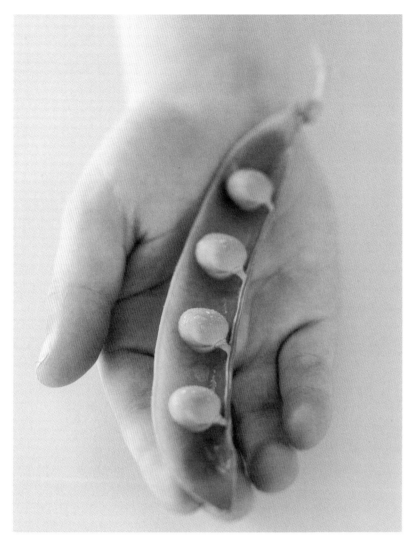

Won't eat...
Peas as a vegetable

Might eat...
Raw mangetout peas in
a salad

Will eat...
Peas in a cheese omelette

Three ways
to get your kids to eat more peas

1 Add peas to salads, stews, casseroles, curries and pasta dishes.

2 Add petit pois to homemade fish cakes or mashed potato.

3 Liven up rice by adding diced peppers, sweetcorn and peas.

Why not try...

Pea and tuna frittata
(see page 36)
Nutritional facts per portion
185 kcal, 11.6 g fat (of which 2.8 g saturates), 1.9 g sugars, 0.4 g salt

Pea and potato filo triangles (see page 36)
Nutritional facts per triangle
40 kcal, 1.5 g fat (of which 0.2 g saturates), 0.5 g sugars, 0 g salt

Beating depression

Peas contain good amounts of vitamins B1 and B3, but are also rich in the B vitamin folate, which may help with teenage anxiety. Research shows that folate levels are often low in depressed people. Peas are an especially good choice for children as they are usually more popular than other folate-containing vegetables such as watercress, spinach and sprouts.

Looking forward

As well as the positive health benefits linked to soluble fibre, peas provide two naturally occurring plant chemicals, lutein and zeaxanthin. These may help reduce the risk of age-related macular degeneration, a leading cause of blindness.

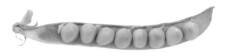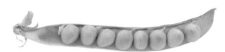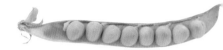

Pea and tuna frittata

● Preparation time **15 mins, plus standing** ● Cooking time **9–12 mins** ● Serves **6**

2 tbsp **mild olive oil**
4 **spring onions, finely sliced**
1 **garlic clove, finely chopped**
2 tbsp **finely diced
  red pepper**
200 g (7 oz) **can tuna
  in water, drained**
300 g (10 oz) **peas (thawed
  if frozen)**
6 **large eggs, lightly beaten**
pepper

1 Heat the oil in a deep, nonstick frying pan over a medium heat. Add the spring onions, garlic and red pepper, stir-fry for 3–4 minutes and then stir in the tuna and peas. Stir to combine and mix well.

2 Season the eggs with pepper and pour over the pea mixture. Cook over a medium heat for 6–8 minutes or until the base of the frittata is set.

3 Remove from the heat and place the frying pan under a preheated grill. Cook the top of the frittata for 3–4 minutes or until set and lightly golden. Remove from the grill and allow to rest for 5–6 minutes. Serve the frittata hot or chilled from the fridge, cut into wedges or squares.

Pea and potato filo triangles

● Preparation time **30 mins, plus cooling** ● Cooking time **18–23 mins** ● Makes **18**

1 tbsp **olive oil,
  plus extra for brushing**
2 **spring onions, finely
  chopped**
200 g (7 oz) **peas (thawed
  if frozen)**
300 g (10 oz) **boiled and
  roughly mashed potatoes**
3 tbsp **finely chopped
  dill or parsley**
3 large sheets of **filo pastry,
  each about 30 x 20 cm
  (12 x 8 inches)**
pepper

1 Heat the oil in a large, nonstick frying pan. Add the spring onions, peas and potatoes and stir-fry for 2–3 minutes until well mixed. Remove from the heat. When cool, stir in the chopped herbs and season with pepper.

2 Working quickly, lay the 3 sheets of filo on top of each other and cut them in half widthways. Cut each half into 3 strips, giving a total of 6 strips of filo per sheet. Lay the filo strips on a clean surface and lightly brush each one with the oil.

3 Place a heaped teaspoon of the pea mixture at the bottom of each strip and fold the pastry diagonally to enclose the filling, forming a sealed triangle. Repeat with the remaining filling and filo strips.

4 Grease and line a large baking sheet and bake in a preheated oven, 190°C (375°F), Gas Mark 5, for 15–20 minutes or until crisp and gold.

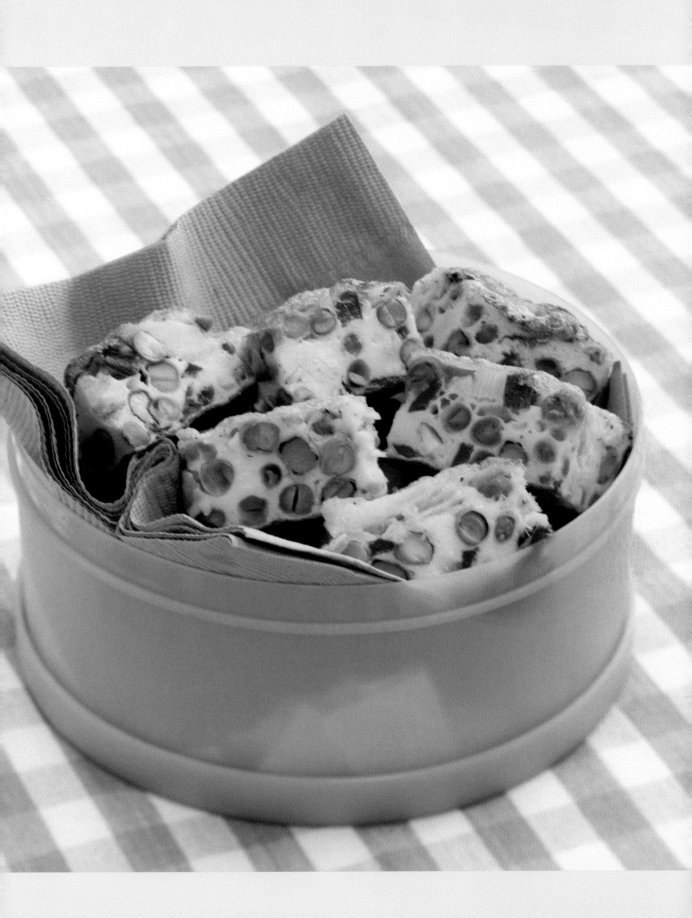

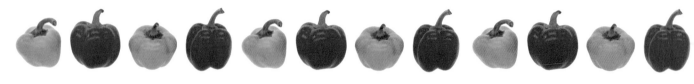

Peppers

Add a rainbow of colours plus plenty of essential vitamins and minerals to your children's meals by including fresh peppers.

What's in them?

Red peppers

Nutrients	100 g (3½ oz)	80 g (a half)
Calories	32 kcal	26 kcal
Protein	1 g	0.8 g
Fat	0.4 g	0.3 g
Carb	6.4 g	5.1 g
Fibre	1.6 g	1.3 g
Vitamin A	640mcg	512 mcg
Vitamin B6	0.4 mg	0.3 mg
Vitamin C	140 mg	112 mg

Benefits

- Help wound healing
- Boost immunity
- Good for joints
- Aid healthy lungs

Pick peppers

Peppers don't just add colour, taste and texture to meals, they are also packed with fibre, beta-carotene, vitamin B6 and vitamin C. They're a great choice for young children because in spite of their name, they're not 'hot' – a recessive gene within them eliminates capsaisin, the compound responsible for the 'hotness' in chilli peppers.

Colourful protection

Different coloured peppers vary in their nutritional content: red peppers contain 14 times more beta-carotene than green ones and are also a good source of the antioxidant lycopene (see Tomatoes); green peppers contain around twice as much folate as red ones. But regardless of the colour, they all contain good amounts of two powerful antioxidants, vitamin C and beta-carotene. These antioxidants work together to destroy harmful free radicals, which damage cells and potentially cause health problems such as heart disease, cancer and asthma.

C it to believe it

Parents might be surprised to learn that peppers are a fantastic source of vitamin C. Just half a red pepper contains more vitamin C than an orange and provides four times the amount needed by children under the age of ten. Quite simply, adding peppers to your child's diet also adds all the health-promoting benefits of vitamin C, which include healing wounds, boosting immunity and helping to prevent asthma (see Oranges).

Good for joints

Peppers are a great choice for children suffering with joint problems. According to the Arthritis Research Campaign, every

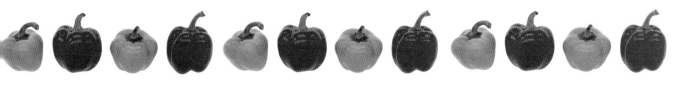

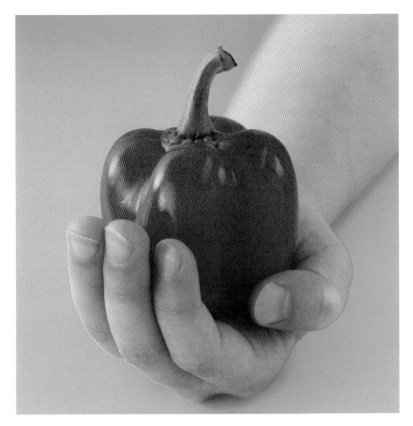

Won't eat...
Raw pepper in salad

Might eat...
Chicken and pepper fajitas

Will eat...
Diced pepper on pizza

Three ways
to get your kids to eat
more peppers

1 Add diced pepper to
pasta sauces, stir-fries
and quiche.

2 Mix finely diced peppers
with tuna, sweetcorn
and a little reduced-fat
mayonnaise and use to fill
baked potatoes, sandwiches
or wraps.

3 Serve raw pepper slices
with a favourite dip.

year around 4 per cent of children under the age of 16 in the UK see their doctor for arthritis or related conditions. Peppers contain the carotenoid beta-cryptoxanthin, which research shows may prevent the inflammation that triggers arthritis.

Healthy lungs

Getting children to eat peppers may help keep their lungs healthy, especially if they are exposed to passive smoke. Research shows that higher levels of beta-cryptoxanthin are associated with improved lung function and a reduced risk of lung cancer, especially in people who smoke or inhale second-hand smoke.

Fat facts

Good news if your children like peppers roasted in olive oil or will only eat them raw with a creamy dip. Fat helps the body to absorb beta-cryptoxanthin. Peppers also contain nutrients that may help prevent heart disease, certain cancers, emphysema and cataracts.

Why not try...
Jewelled couscous (see page 40)
Nutritional facts per portion
181 kcal, 8.1 g fat (of which 1.1 g saturates), 6.5 g sugars, 0 g salt

Oriental grilled vegetable sticks (see page 40)
Nutritional facts per stick
47 kcal, 2.8 g fat (of which 0.4 g saturates), 4.6 g sugars, 0.2 g salt

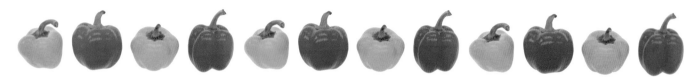

Jewelled couscous

● Preparation time **30 mins, plus standing** ● Cooking time **15–20 mins** ● Serves **6**

4 tbsp **olive oil**
2 **peppers (red and yellow),**
    cored, deseeded and cut
    into 1.5 cm (¾ inch) pieces
200 g (7 oz) **cherry tomatoes**
1 **courgette, cut into 1.5 cm**
    (¾ inch) pieces
1 large **red onion, cut into**
    1.5 cm (¾ inch) pieces
200 g (7 oz) **couscous**
2–3 tbsp **chopped mixed**
herbs (such as parsley, mint
    and coriander)
pepper

1 Grease and line 2 large baking sheets. Place all the vegetables in a large mixing bowl and add the olive oil. Toss to mix well, season with pepper and spread this mixture in a single layer on the baking sheets. Roast in a preheated oven, 200°C (400°F), Gas Mark 6, for 15–20 minutes or until lightly browned at the edges.

2 Meanwhile, place the couscous in a large mixing bowl and pour over boiling water to just cover. Cover with clingfilm and allow to stand for 10–15 minutes, until all the liquid has been absorbed. Uncover and fluff up the couscous grains with a fork.

3 Transfer to a shallow serving dish. Add the roasted vegetables together with the roasting juices to the couscous and stir to mix well. Stir in the chopped herbs and serve immediately.

Oriental grilled vegetable sticks

● Preparation time **15 mins, plus marinating** ● Cooking time **6–8 mins** ● Makes **8**

1 **red pepper, cored,**
    deseeded and cut into
    12 pieces
1 **yellow pepper, cored,**
    deseeded and cut into
    12 pieces
4 **cherry tomatoes**
2 **spring onions, each cut**
    into 4 pieces
1 tsp **toasted sesame oil**
1 **garlic clove, crushed**
1 tbsp **reduced-salt soy sauce**
1 tbsp **clear honey**
1 tbsp **olive oil**

1 Put the vegetables in a mixing bowl. Mix together the sesame oil, garlic, soy sauce, honey and oil and pour over the vegetables. Toss to mix well, cover and marinate for 1–2 hours in the fridge.

2 Thread the vegetables on to 8 metal or presoaked bamboo skewers, so that each skewer has an even mixture of all the vegetables.

3 Place under a preheated grill and cook for 6–8 minutes, turning once and brushing with any reserved marinade.

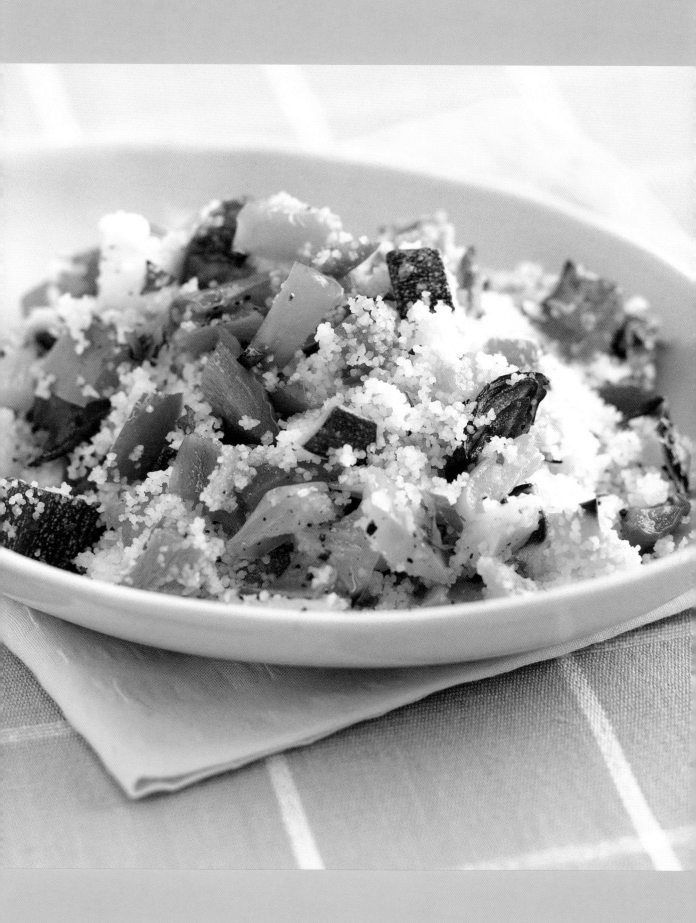

Tomatoes

What's in them?

Raw tomatoes

Nutrients	100 g (3½ oz)	85 g (1 tomato)
Calories	17 kcal	14 kcal
Protein	0.7 g	0.6 g
Fat	0.3 g	0.3 g
Carb	3.1 g	2.6 g
Fibre	1 g	0.9 g
Vitamin A	94 mcg	80 mcg
Vitamin C	17 mg	14 mg
Vitamin E	1.2 mg	1 mg

Benefits

- Prevents cancer
- Eases asthma
- Sun protection

Great in soups, salads, pizzas and pasta, with their good selection of nutrients, tomatoes are also a key ingredient for keeping kids healthy.

You say tomato

Tomatoes are packed with health-promoting beta-carotene and vitamins C and E. But the real health hero is lycopene, a disease-fighting plant chemical that gives tomatoes their red colour and acts as an antioxidant. As well as preventing cancer, lycopene may also ease asthma and protect the skin from sunburn.

Prevent cancer

Research shows that lycopene may protect against cancer of the prostate, lung, digestive system and breast, so encouraging your kids to eat tomatoes regularly could prevent these diseases in adulthood. According to studies, eating good amounts of tomatoes halves the risk of stomach cancer and reduces the risk of colon and rectal cancers by 60 per cent. And getting boys into the tomato-eating habit is particularly important as five studies suggest that good intakes of lycopene reduce the risk of prostate cancer by 30 to 40 per cent.

Ease the wheeze

Both beta-carotene (see Carrots) and vitamin C (see Oranges), which are found in tomatoes, have been linked to reducing the symptoms of asthma. But research also shows that lycopene may help ease asthma brought on by exercising. Indeed, a study in the *European Respiratory Journal* found that tomatoes protected against wheezing and shortness of breath in 6–7-year-olds. More research is needed, but encouraging asthmatic children to eat tomatoes certainly won't do any harm.

Sun protection

Tomatoes may help to protect children from the harmful effects of the sun. Research shows that lycopene accumulates in the

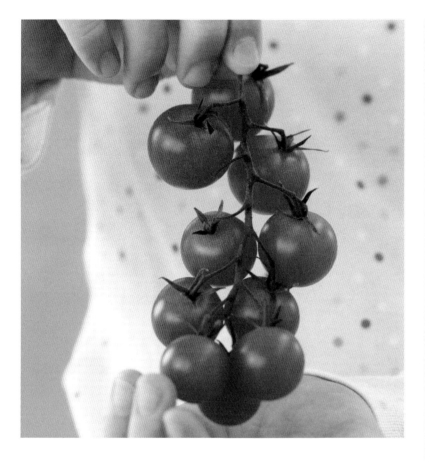

skin where its antioxidant properties potentially help to
reduce the damaging effects of ultraviolet light. Far more
research needs to be carried out to confirm these findings and
it's unlikely that eating tomatoes will ever replace traditional
sun-protection methods such as covering up and wearing sun
screen with a high SPF. But a few cherry tomatoes with a
picnic won't do any harm.

Go for the squash

Don't panic if ketchup, pasta sauce and pizza are the only way
to get tomatoes into your kids. Cooked tomatoes are a more
concentrated source of lycopene, and the body is better able to
absorb it. Adding fat boosts the absorption of lycopene further –
a perfect reason to add cheese to pizzas and pasta dishes.

Looking forward

As well as helping to protect against cancer, tomatoes may also
help to prevent heart disease thanks to their lycopene content.

Won't eat...
Tomatoes in salad

Might eat...
A bowl of tomato soup

Will eat...
Pasta with tomato sauce
and grated cheese

Three ways
to get your kids to eat
more tomatoes

1 Add a handful of
cherry tomatoes to
packed lunches.

2 Top toast or bagels with
grilled lean bacon and
sliced tomato for a nutritious
breakfast.

3 Use plenty of canned
tomatoes, passatta and
tomato purée in cooking.

Why not try...

Scrummy tomato sauce
(see page 44)
Nutritional facts per portion
21 kcal, 2.9 g fat (of which
0.45 saturates), 5.8 g sugars,
0.1 g salt

Rich tomato and cannellini spread
(see page 44)
Nutritional facts per portion
258 kcal, 5.9 g fat (of which 0.9 g
saturates), 6.6 g sugars, 0.9 g salt

Scrummy pasta and tomato sauce

● Preparation time **20 mins** ● Cooking time **30–35 mins** ● Serves **6**

1 tbsp **olive oil**
1 **small onion, finely chopped**
3 **garlic cloves, finely chopped**
2 **celery sticks, finely chopped**
1 **carrot, finely chopped**
1 tsp **ground cinnamon**
400 g (13 oz) **can chopped tomatoes**
1 **bay leaf**
1 tsp **golden caster sugar**
2 tbsp **finely chopped basil**
300 g **fusili pasta**
pepper

1 Heat the oil in a medium-sized, heavy-based saucepan. Add the onion, garlic, celery and carrot, stir and cook over a gentle heat for 6–8 minutes or until the vegetables have softened.

2 Add the cinnamon, tomatoes, bay leaf, sugar and basil and season with pepper. Bring to the boil, cover, reduce the heat to cook for 20–25 minutes, stirring occasionally, until thickened and glossy. If you want a thinner sauce add a little water.

3 While the sauce is simmering, cook the pasta according to the packet instructions. Drain and serve with the tomato sauce.

Rich tomato and cannellini spread

● Preparation time **10 mins** ● Cooking time **12–15 mins** ● Serves **6**

4 **plum tomatoes, halved**
2 tbsp **olive oil**
200 g (7 oz) **can cannellini beans in water, drained and rinsed**
2 **garlic cloves, crushed**
1 tsp **balsamic vinegar**
1 tsp **clear honey**
2 tbsp **finely chopped flat leaf parsley**
3–4 tbsp **lemon juice**
pepper
6 **English muffins or wholegrain toast, to serve**

1 Grease and line a baking sheet. Toss the tomatoes with the oil and place them, cut side up, on the baking sheet. Season with pepper and roast in a preheated oven, 200°C (400°F), Gas Mark 6, for 12–15 minutes.

2 Remove from the oven and transfer to a food processor or blender with all the pan juices. Add the beans to the tomatoes and then the garlic, balsamic vinegar, honey, parsley and lemon juice. Process until fairly smooth. Serve with English muffins or wholegrain toast.

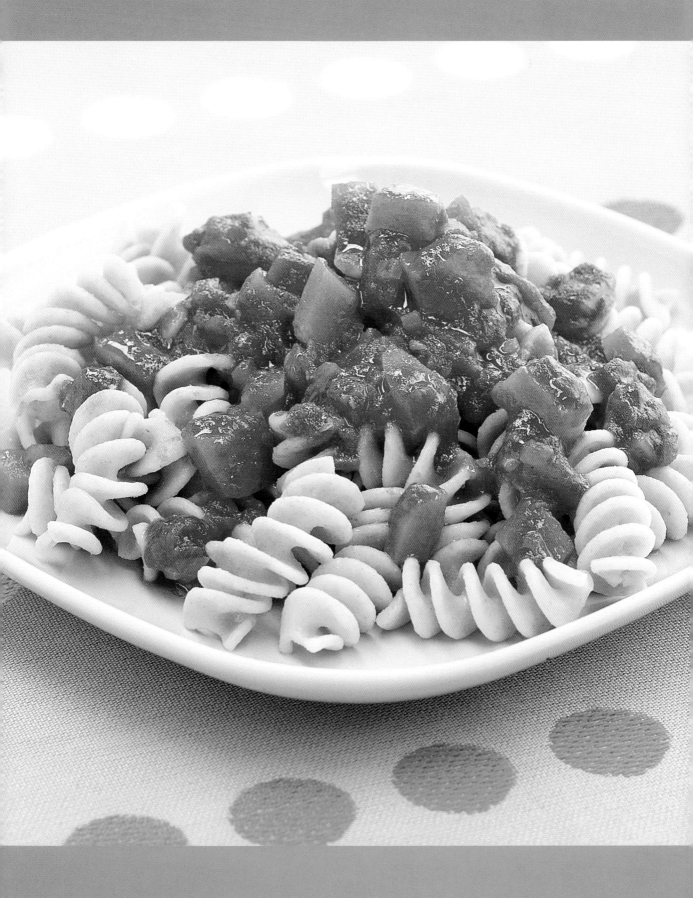

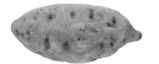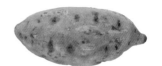

Sweet potato

What's in it?
Boiled sweet potato

Nutrients	100 g (3½ oz)	65 g (Each)
Calories	76 kcal	49 kcal
Protein	1.4 g	0.9 g
Fat	0.1 g	0.1 g
Carb	17.7 g	11.5 g
Fibre	2.5 g	1.6 g
Vitamin A	1,574 mcg	1,023 mcg
Vitamin C	13 mg	8 mg
Vitamin E	0.9 mg	0.6 mg

Benefits
- Prevents obesity and diabetes
- Prevents constipation
- Helps eyesight
- Great for a sweet tooth

Keep your kids sweet and healthy – top up their antioxidant levels by switching normal spuds for sweet potatoes from time to time.

Spuds they'll like

This is one sweet food you can encourage kids to eat. According to America's Center for Science in the Public Interest, sweet potatoes top the list when compared with the nutritional value of all other vegetables. It's not surprising considering that they are packed with fibre and antioxidants beta-carotene and vitamins C and E.

Fill up the fat-free way

Sweet potatoes contain fibre, so are a great choice for hungry children. As well as keeping the digestive system healthy and preventing constipation, fibre is filling and can help control children's appetites. Unlike regular spuds, sweet potatoes also have a low glycaemic index and so keep blood-sugar levels low and steady. As well as preventing mood swings, this can keep the munchies at bay, helping to stop children from becoming overweight.

Prevent diabetes

If you have a family history of diabetes, add sweet potatoes to mealtimes. New research suggests that carotenoids in foods such as sweet potatoes may help to prevent insulin resistance, a pre-curser to diabetes.

Satisfy a sweet tooth

Sweet potatoes are a great choice for sweet-toothed children. Research shows that children prefer a sweeter taste than adults. But to keep teeth, waistlines and taste buds happy, encourage kids to get their sugar fix from naturally sweet foods such as sweet potatoes, rather than sweets, chocolate and biscuits that contain few other nutrients.

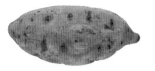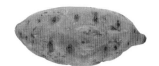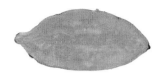

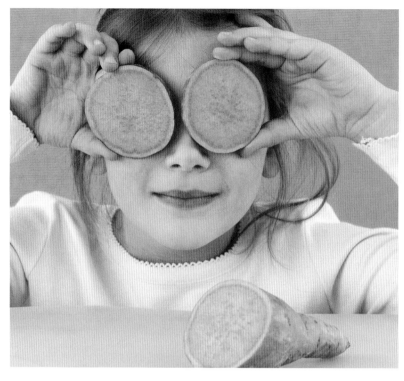

Boost vitamin A

Switching spuds for sweet potatoes may boost vitamin A intakes, a nutrient often lacking in children's diets (see Carrots). One study found that vitamin A stores were significantly higher in children given orange-fleshed sweet potatoes than those given white-fleshed sweet potatoes. The magic ingredient is beta-carotene, which gives sweet potatoes their orange colour and is used by the body to make vitamin A.

A new vision

Research shows just how important beta-carotene can be for children's eyes. In Africa, scientists are encouraging mothers to cook with orange-fleshed sweet potatoes rather than traditional white ones in an effort to prevent blindness, which affects around three million African under-fives and is caused by a lack of vitamin A.

Looking forward

The antioxidants in sweet potatoes may help to prevent heart disease, certain cancers and inflammatory conditions such as osteoarthritis and asthma.

Won't eat...
Boiled sweet potato

Might eat...
Sweet potato mashed with regular potato

Will eat...
Sweet potato wedges

Three ways
to get your kids to eat more sweet potato

1 Add chunks of sweet potato to casseroles and stews.

2 Roast sweet potatoes with parsnips and carrots in olive oil.

3 Use sweet potato in place of regular potatoes. For example, try baked sweet potatoes or sweet potato chips.

Why not try...
Sweet potato risotto
(see page 48)
Nutritional facts per portion
260 kcal, 5.2 g fat (of which 0.9 g saturates), 3.3 g sugars, 0.1 g salt

Roasted sweet potato soup
(see page 48)
Nutritional facts per portion
102 kcal, 2.3 g fat (of which 0.4 g saturates), 7.2 g sugars, 0.1 g salt

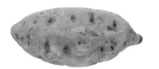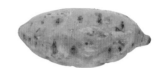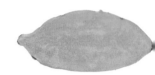

Sweet potato risotto

● Preparation time **15 mins** ● Cooking time **30–35 mins** ● Serves **6**

2 tbsp **olive oil**
1 **onion, finely chopped**
2 **garlic cloves, finely chopped**
200 g (7 oz) **sweet potato, cut into 1.5 cm (¾ inch) dice**
300 g (10 oz) **arborio rice**
750 ml (1¼ pint) **hot homemade, salt-free vegetable or chicken stock**
2–3 tbsp **finely chopped flat leaf parsley**
pepper
grated Parmesan cheese

1. Heat the oil in a large, heavy-based saucepan. Add the onion and garlic and cook, stirring, over a gentle heat until the onion has softened. Add the sweet potato and rice and stir for a further 1–2 minutes to mix well.

2. Turn the heat to medium and add a ladleful of the hot stock. Stir and cook gently until all the liquid has been absorbed and then add another ladleful of stock. Continue cooking the risotto in this manner, stirring constantly and adding the stock until the rice is creamy and just tender to the bite. This should take 20–25 minutes.

3. Remove the pan from the heat, stir in the parsley and season with pepper. Stir to mix well, sprinkle over the grated Parmesan and serve.

Roasted sweet potato soup

● Preparation time **20 mins, plus cooling** ● Cooking time **55–65 mins** ● Serves **6**

2 **sweet potatoes, about 250 g (8 oz) each**
1 tbsp **olive oil**
6 **spring onions, finely sliced**
1 **garlic clove, crushed**
1 **large carrot, roughly chopped**
1 **bay leaf**
pinch of **sweet pimenton or paprika**
1 tsp **ground cumin**
1 tsp **ground cinnamon**
600 ml (1 pint) **homemade, salt-free vegetable or chicken stock**
wholemeal croutons or bread, to serve

1. Place the sweet potatoes on a nonstick baking sheet and roast them in a preheated oven, 200°C (400°F), Gas Mark 6, for 25–30 minutes. Remove and allow to cool before cutting each one in half and scooping out the flesh. Set aside.

2. Heat the oil in a medium-sized saucepan. Add the spring onions, garlic and carrot, stir-fry for 2–3 minutes over a medium heat and then add the bay leaf, pimenton or paprika, cumin and cinnamon.

3. Stir and cook for 1–2 minutes and then add the sweet potato flesh and stock. Bring the mixture to the boil, stir well, reduce the heat to low, cover and simmer gently for 25–30 minutes, stirring occasionally.

4. Remove from the heat and use a hand-held electric whisk or a blender to process the soup until smooth. (For a thinner soup add more stock.) Serve with wholemeal croutons or bread.

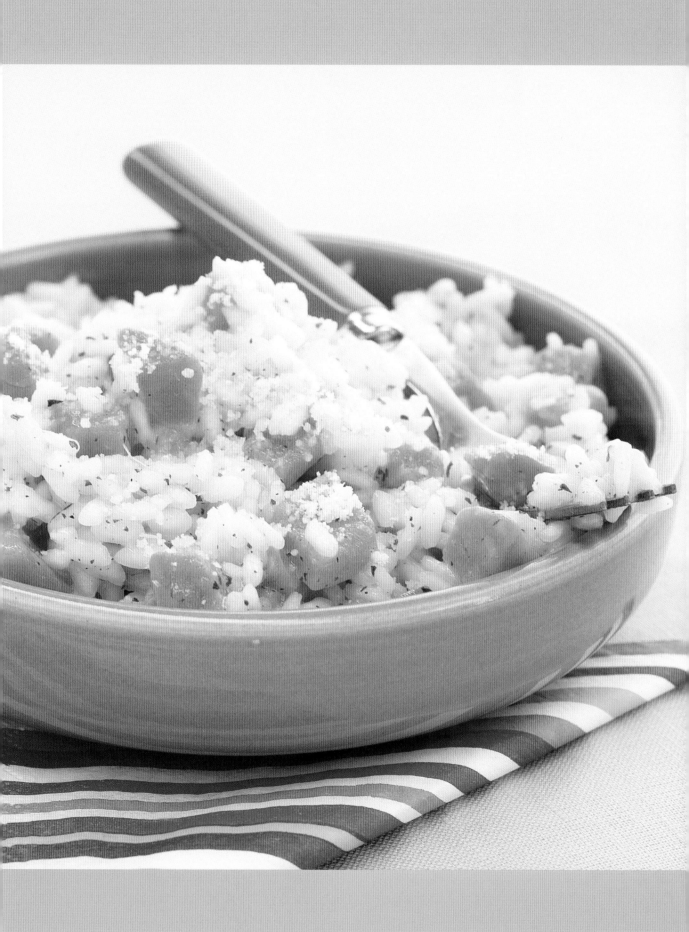

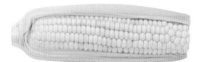 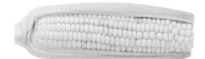 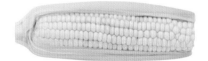

Sweetcorn

What's in it?
Canned sweetcorn

Nutrients	100 g (3½ oz)	30g (1 tbsp)
Calories	122 kcal	37 kcal
Protein	2.9 g	0.9 g
Fat	1.2 g	0.4 g
Carb	26.6 g	8 g
Fibre	1.4 g	0.4 g

Benefits
- Helps prevent constipation
- Combats diabetes
- Weight control
- Beats heart disease and cancer

Whether topping pizzas with sweetcorn or having baby corn with a dip, adding this vegetable to your child's diet is a sweet way to keep them healthy.

Sweet nutrients
The sweet taste of this vegetable makes it a hit with children. But parents should love it too, because it is packed with fibre, which can prevent constipation, a common complaint in young children.

The whole story
Most kids and parents may think that sweetcorn is simply another vegetable, but this superfood is also a wholegrain. This means it has the same health benefits as brown rice, wholemeal pasta, wholemeal bread, oats and rye. All the components in wholegrains – fibre, antioxidants, vitamins, minerals, complex carbohydrates and phytonutrients – work together to prevent disease. Health experts agree that from five years of age onwards, everyone should eat five daily servings of fruit and vegetables and three daily servings of wholegrains. Eating sweetcorn fulfils both these recommendations at the same time: six baby corn, three heaped tablespoons of sweetcorn kernels or one corn-on-the-cob counts as one serving of vegetable AND one serving of wholegrains.

Preventing diabetes
Type 2 diabetes, which was typically seen in people over 40 years of age, is increasingly being diagnosed in children, usually as a result of obesity. Eating more wholegrains such sweetcorn can help prevent this disease. A study in the *American Journal of Epidemiology* found that teenagers who ate more than 1.5 servings of wholegrains daily were more sensitive to the effects of insulin, had a lower body-mass index and a smaller waist circumference than those who ate less than half a serving daily. This is beneficial as insulin resistance and obesity are precursors of Type 2 diabetes.

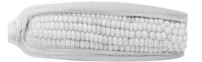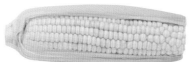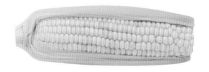

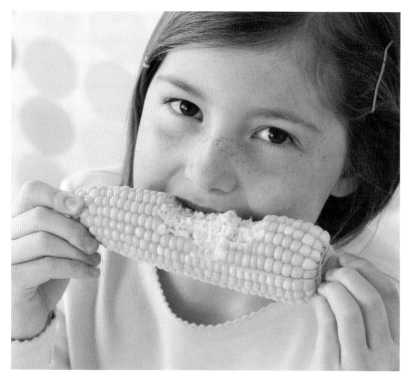

Fill up on antioxidants

Getting children to eat antioxidant-rich fruit and vegetables isn't always easy, so it's good news if you can encourage them to munch on sweetcorn. Research from Cornell University in the US shows that sweetcorn contains more antioxidants than many other fruits, vegetables and other wholegrains, with twice the antioxidant activity of broccoli, spinach, wholewheat and oats, and more than three times the activity of brown rice.

Can be good for you

Don't panic if your kids will only eat canned sweetcorn. More research from Cornell University reveals that the heat treatment used to process sweetcorn increases its antioxidant activity further, giving it even more health benefits. But opt for varieties canned without added sugar or salt.

Looking forward

More than 50 scientific studies have shown that consuming wholegrain foods regularly reduces the risk of heart disease and certain cancers by up to 30 per cent. And numerous studies show that eating more wholegrains helps prevent diabetes and obesity.

Won't eat...
Sweetcorn as a vegetable

Might eat...
Baby corn with a dip

Will eat...
A tuna and sweetcorn sandwich

Three ways
to get your kids to eat more sweetcorn

1 Add canned or frozen sweetcorn to soups, pasta and rice dishes.

2 Top pizza with sweetcorn.

3 Add baby corn to stir-fries and salads.

Why not try...
Skillet corn bread
(see page 52)

Nutritional facts per slice
268 kcal, 12.3 g fat (of which 2.3 g saturates), 3.2 g sugars, 0.4 g salt

Quick chicken, mushroom and sweetcorn chowder
(see page 52)

Nutritional facts per portion
109 kcal, 2.1 g fat (of which 0.4 g saturates), 1.3 g sugars, 0.1 g salt

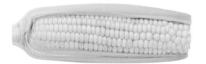
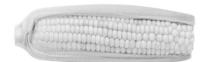
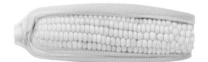

Skillet corn bread

● Preparation time **15 mins** ● Cooking time **20–25 mins** ● Makes **8 wedges**

60 g (2¼ oz) **plain flour**
175 g (6 oz) **coarse cornmeal or polenta**
1½ tsp **baking powder**
1 tsp **golden caster sugar**
1 tsp **ground cinnamon**
3 **large eggs, lightly beaten**
60 ml (2¼ fl oz) **olive oil**
100 ml (3¼ fl oz) **buttermilk**
200 ml (7 fl oz) **milk**
250 g (8 oz) **fresh, canned or thawed sweetcorn kernels, drained**

1 Put the flour, cornmeal, baking powder, sugar and cinnamon in a large bowl and mix together.

2 Put the eggs, olive oil, buttermilk and milk in a separate bowl and whisk until smooth. Beat this mixture into the dry ingredients with the sweetcorn and stir until thoroughly combined.

3 Lightly grease a 25 cm (10 inch) cake tin and pour in the dough mixture. Level the surface and bake in a preheated oven, 190°C (375°F), Gas Mark 5, for 20–25 minutes or until the bread has risen and is lightly browned and a skewer, inserted into the centre, comes out clean.

4 Remove from the oven and allow to stand for 4–5 minutes before cutting into wedges. Serve immediately.

Quick chicken, mushroom & sweetcorn chowder

● Preparation time **15 mins** ● Cooking time **about 10 mins** ● Serves **6**

800 ml (28 fl oz) **homemade, salt-free chicken or vegetable stock**
200 g (7 oz) **cooked chicken, skinned and cut into 1 cm (½ inch) dice**
250 g (8 oz) **chestnut mushrooms, finely chopped**
325 g (11 oz) **fresh, canned or thawed sweetcorn kernels, drained**
3 **spring onions, finely sliced**
2 tbsp **finely chopped dill (optional)**
pepper

1 Put the stock in a saucepan and bring to the boil. Add the chicken, mushrooms and sweetcorn and bring back to the boil. Reduce the heat to medium and simmer gently for 5–6 minutes.

2 Stir in the spring onions and season with pepper. Remove from the heat, stir in the dill (if used) and serve immediately.

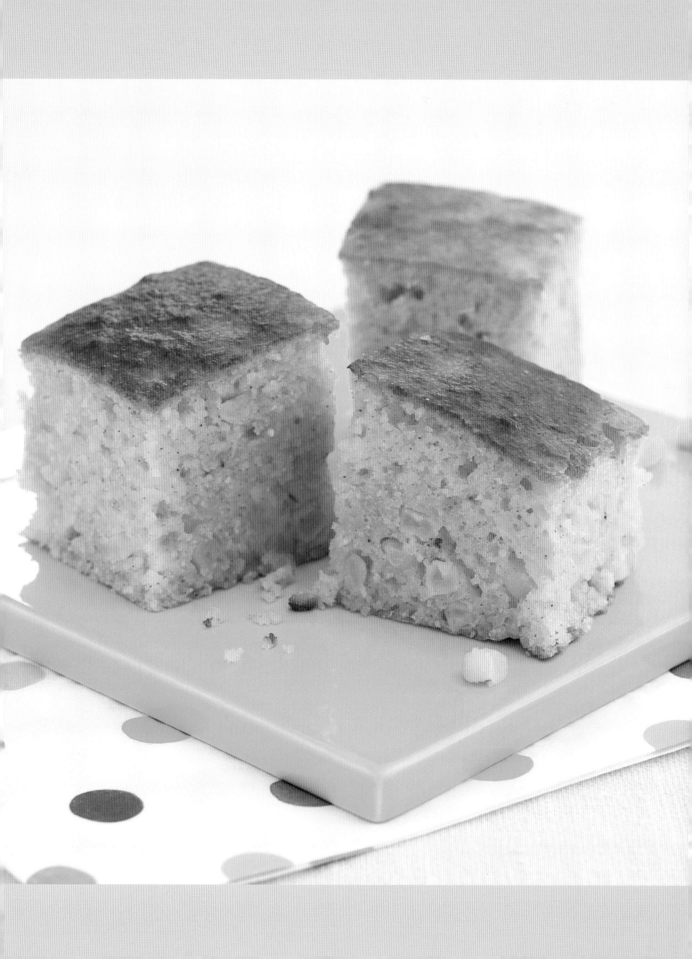

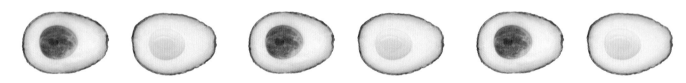

Avocado

It's not just children's hearts that will love it if they eat avocado. This nutrient-rich fruit has many other health benefits for growing bodies.

What's in them?
Avocado

Nutrients	100 g (3½ oz)	50g ½ a small avocado
Calories	190 kcal	95 kcal
Protein	1.9 g	1 g
Fat	19.5 g	9.8 g
Carb	1.9 g	1 g
Fibre	3.4 g	1.7 g
Vitamin B6	0.4 mg	0.2 mg
Vitamin E	3.2 mg	1.6 mg
Potassium	450 mg	225 mg
Copper	0.2 mg	0.1 mg

Benefits

- Nutrient-rich for small tummies
- Good fats to fight heart disease
- Boosts nutrients from other vegetables
- Good for skin

Great for growing kids

Avocados contain good amounts of fibre, potassium, copper and vitamins B6 and E. They are also high in fat (and therefore calories), but most of these fats are heart-healthy monounsaturates. This makes avocados especially good for young children who have small tummies and need lots of nutrients and calories in a small amount of food.

Balancing fats

Children under the age of five should not have a low-fat diet (see Introduction), but it is important that the fats they do eat come from nutrient-rich foods such as avocado. After five years old, children should switch to a diet that is low in total fat and saturates. Unfortunately, figures from the last National Diet and Nutrition Survey of Young People show that, on average, children get more than 14 per cent of their calories from saturates rather than the recommended 11 per cent. In contrast, less than 12 per cent of their calories come from monounsaturates rather than the recommended 13 per cent. Switching less healthy saturate-rich foods for those rich in monounsaturates will improve the balance of fats in your child's diet, helping to prevent heart disease in later life. So start by topping salads with avocado rather than mayonnaise.

Nutrient booster

Add avocado to salads or salsa and your child will get more out of their vegetables. Research shows the fat in avocado increases the body's ability to absorb health-promoting carotenoids such as beta-carotene (see Carrots) and lycopene (see Tomatoes) from salad vegetables. Full-fat dressings have the same effect, but unlike avocados, they often contain few other nutrients.

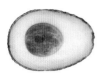

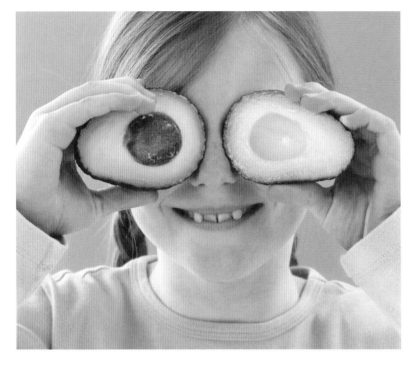

A potassium punch

Avocados are packed with potassium, which controls heartbeat and blood pressure, and works with sodium to regulate fluid balance – just one small avocado contains more potassium than a banana. Eating fewer salty foods and more potassium-rich foods can help prevent high blood pressure. So why not provide hungry teenagers with homemade guacamole and pitta instead of potato crisps after school?

Healthy skin

Getting kids to eat avocado may help to improve skin complaints such as acne and eczema, thanks to their vitamin E content. This nutrient helps skin heal and prevents scarring, making it especially important for children who frequently cut or bruise themselves.

Looking forward

As well as containing heart-healthy monounsaturates, avocado contains beta-sitosterol and glutathione, which help prevent heart disease and cancer. Avocado also contains cancer-fighting vitamin E and lutein, an antioxidant that also protects against eye diseases.

Won't eat...
Avocado in a salad

Might eat...
Avocado dip with pitta bread

Will eat...
Chicken fajitas with homemade guacamole

Three ways
to get your kids to eat more avocado

1 Top baked potatoes with avocado, tomato and lemon juice.

2 Use mashed avocado in sandwiches in place of mayonnaise, butter or spread.

3 For an after-school snack, fill pitta breads with avocado, tomatoes and mozzarella cheese.

Why not try...

Avocado dip with roasted potato wedges
(see page 56)
Nutritional facts per portion
190 kcal, 14 g fat (of which 2.9 g saturates), 1.4 g sugars, 0 g salt

Avocado, mozzarella, tomato and pasta salad
(see page 56)
Nutritional facts per portion
323 kcal, 24.1 g fat (of which 8 g saturates), 5 g sugars, 0.4 g salt

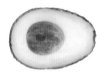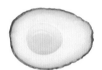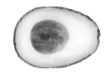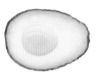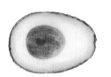

Avocado dip with roasted potato wedges

● Preparation time **30 mins** ● Cooking time **20–25 mins** ● Serves **6**

Wedges
2 **large baking potatoes**
olive oil, to brush
mild paprika, to sprinkle
ground cumin, to sprinkle
Dip
2 **ripe avocados**
juice of 1 **lime**
1 **garlic clove, crushed**
2 tbsp **extra virgin olive oil**
2–3 tbsp **finely chopped**
   fresh coriander leaves
1 **plum tomato, deseeded**
   and finely chopped
1 tbsp **finely chopped**
   red onion
2 tsp **finely chopped cucumber**
pepper
mixed vegetable sticks,
   to serve

1 Grease and line a baking sheet. Cut the potatoes into long wedges and arrange them on the baking sheet in a single layer. Brush lightly with olive oil and sprinkle over the paprika and cumin. Bake in a preheated oven, 200°C (400°F), Gas Mark 6, for 20–25 minutes or until golden-brown and tender.

2 Meanwhile, make the dip. Halve the avocados, discard the stones and scoop the flesh into a food processor or blender with the lime juice, garlic and olive oil. Process until smooth and transfer the purée to a bowl. Fold in the coriander, tomato, onion and cucumber and season with pepper.

3 Place the avocado dip in the centre of a large platter and surround with the potato wedges. Serve accompanied with carrot sticks, celery sticks and sliced red and green peppers.

Avocado, mozzarella, tomato and pasta salad

● Preparation time **20 mins** ● Cooking time **about 10 mins** ● Serves **6**

100 g (3½ oz) **pasta (such as**
   penne or farfalle)
2 **ripe avocados**
100 g (3½ oz) **mozzarella**
   cheese, drained
4 **ripe plum tomatoes**
½ **small cucumber**
Dressing
4 tbsp **extra virgin olive oil**
juice of 1 **orange**
1 tsp **clear honey**
1 tbsp **balsamic vinegar**
pepper

1 Cook the pasta according to the instructions on the packet, drain and rinse under cold water, drain again and set aside in a large, shallow salad bowl.

2 Make the dressing. Put all the ingredients in a screw-top jar and shake to mix well. Pour over the pasta.

3 Peel, stone and cut the avocados into bite-sized pieces. Cut the mozzarella, tomatoes and cucumber into 1 cm (½ inch) dice. Add to the pasta. Toss to mix well and serve.

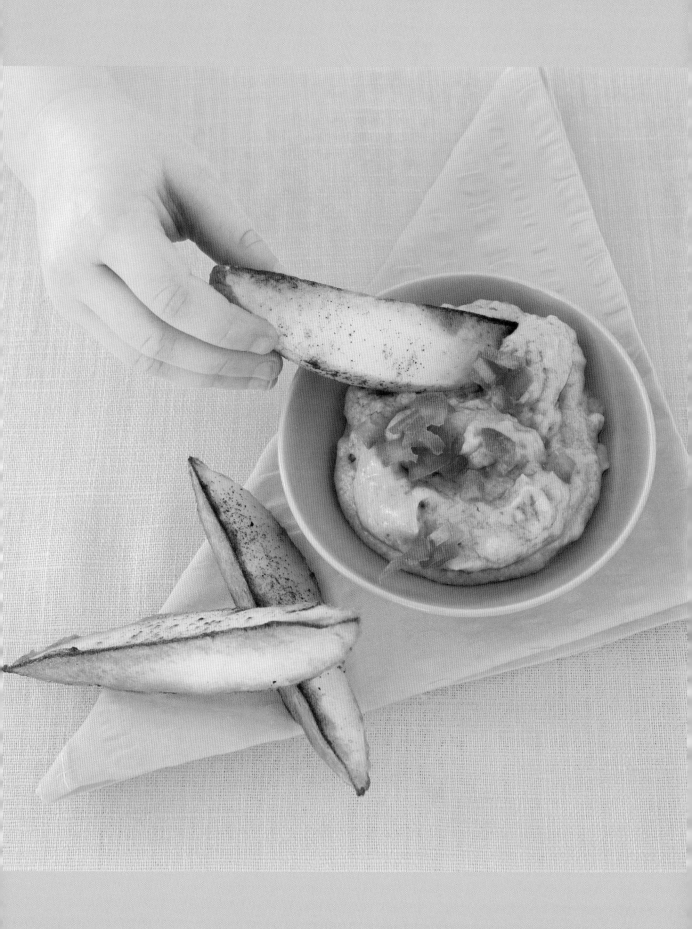

Melon

What's in them?
Cantaloupe melon

Nutrient	100 g (3½ oz)	Per 150 g (5 oz slice)
Calories	19 kcal	29 kcal
Protein	0.6 g	0.9 g
Fat	0.1 g	0.2 g
Carb	4.2 g	6.3 g
Fibre	1 g	1.5 g
Vitamin A	294 mcg	441 mcg
Vitamin C	26 mg	39 mg
Potassium	210 mg	315 mg

Benefits
- Great for skin
- Contributes to fluid intake
- May protect against cancer and heart disease

They are sweet, juicy and refreshing to eat, but those aren't the only reasons for putting melon on the menu for your children.

A colourful fruit
With so many different varieties, colours and textures to choose from, melon is guaranteed to be a hit with children. But it's not just the taste and appearance that makes it such a great choice. These delicious fruits contain potassium and vitamin C (see Oranges), and depending on the variety, may also be packed with beta-carotene (see Carrots). Melon is also a great way to boost fluid intakes in children.

Flesh that's best
The darker the flesh, the more nutrients the melon contains which means that honeydews are usually at the bottom of the nutrient pile, while cantaloupes are at the top. Cantaloupe melon contains 15 times more beta-carotene than watermelon and 37 times more than honeydew. Meanwhile, watermelon is the only variety packed with lycopene, an antioxidant also found in tomatoes that may help prevent certain cancers (see Tomatoes).

Great for skin
Eating more melon could be the perfect beauty boost for teenage girls. Thanks to its high water content, melon helps to keep skin hydrated so it looks smooth and soft. Plus, cantaloupe melon is packed with beta-carotene, which the body uses to make vitamin A, a nutrient essential for healthy skin. There is even some evidence that beta-carotene helps reduce sensitivity to the sun, although more research is needed to confirm this.

Beat dehydration
All melons contain around 92 per cent water. This makes them a great food for helping to prevent dehydration. Children's bodies are three-quarters water, and they require constant

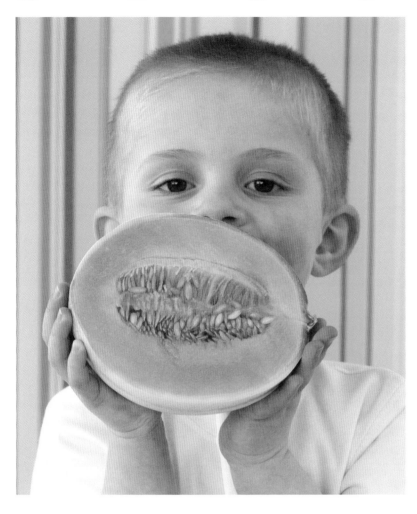

hydration in order to regulate organs, control body temperature and dissolve solids. Furthermore, around 85 per cent of the brain is water, explaining why even mild dehydration causes headaches, lethargy, dizziness and an inability to concentrate – all of which can affect performance at school. Although children need at least six glasses of water a day – more when it's hot or when they've been exercising – foods such as melon can contribute to fluid intakes. A 150 g (5 oz) slice of melon, for example, provides almost 140 ml (4 ½ fl oz) water – a small glassful.

Looking forward

The different antioxidants and vitamin C in melons may prevent cancers and heart disease, while potassium may help to control blood pressure.

Won't eat...
A slice of melon

Might eat...
Melon in a fruit salad

Will eat...
Homemade melon sorbet

Three ways
to get your kids to eat more melon

1 Make your own melon granita – blend melon, lemon juice, ice cubes and a little sugar, then freeze until the mixture becomes a firm slush.

2 Add small chunks of melon to salads.

3 Fill packed lunch boxes with small cubes of cheese and melon on cocktail sticks.

Why not try...

Melon, cucumber and prawn skewers (see page 60)
Nutritional facts per skewer
22 kcal, 0.2 g fat (of which 0 g saturates), 1.9 g sugars, 0.1 g salt

Lunchbox mixed melon salad (see page 60)
Nutritional facts per portion
40 kcal, 0.2 g fat (of which 0 g saturates), 9.2 g sugars, 0.1 g salt

Melon, cucumber and prawn skewers

● Preparation time **10 mins** ● Cooking time **5–6 mins** ● Makes **8**

16 **raw tiger prawns, peeled and deveined**
300 g (10 oz) **charentais melon, peeled and deseeded**
200 g (7 oz) **cucumber**
juice of 1 **lime**
1 tbsp **finely chopped dill (optional)**

1 Place the prawns in a small saucepan of boiling water and cook for 5–6 minutes or until they turn pink and are cooked through. Drain and set aside to cool.

2 Cut the melon and cucumber into 1 cm (½ inch) pieces. Place them in a shallow bowl and add the prawns.

3 Squeeze over the lime juice and sprinkle over the dill (if used). Toss to mix well. To serve, thread the melon, cucumber and prawns evenly on to 8 wooden or presoaked bamboo skewers.

Lunchbox mixed melon salad

● Preparation time **15 mins, plus chilling** ● Serves **6**

300 g (10 oz) **galia melon, peeled and deseeded**
300 g (10 oz) **cantaloupe melon, peeled and deseeded**
300 g (10 oz) **watermelon, peeled and deseeded**
1 large **orange**
mint leaves, to garnish

1 Cut the flesh of the three types of melon into bite-sized pieces or use a melon baller to cut it into balls. Place them in a shallow dish.

2 Halve the orange and squeeze out the juice, discarding any seeds. Pour this over the mixed melon and toss gently to mix well. Cover and chill until ready to eat. Garnish with mint leaves and serve.

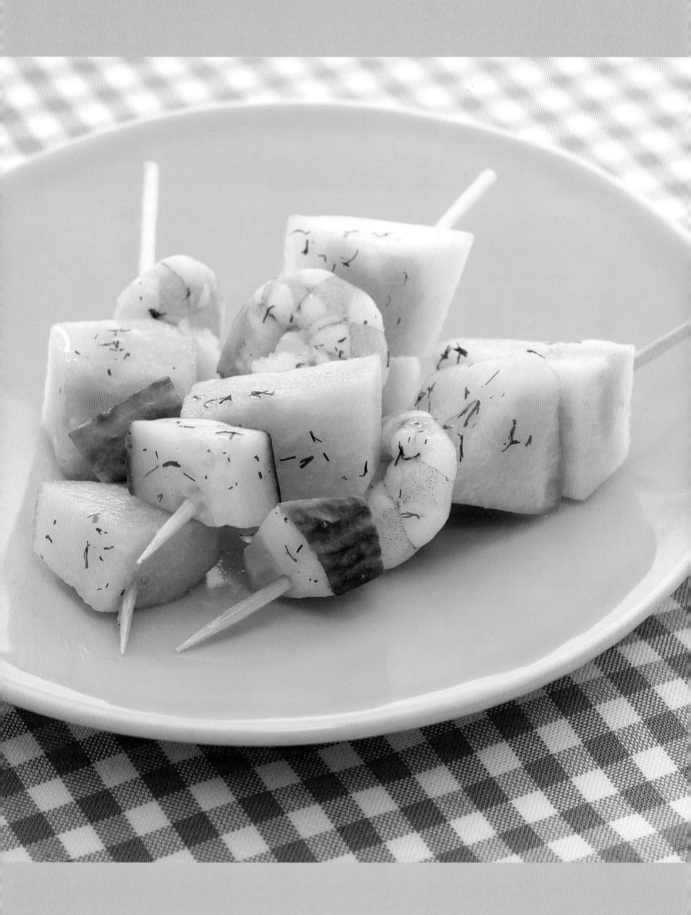

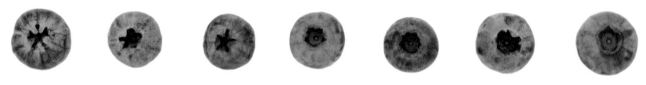

Blueberries

Delicious in cakes, bakes and shakes, blueberries are a great choice for children of all ages and have an impressive range of health benefits.

What's in them?
Blueberries

Nutrient	100 g (3½ oz)	50 g/2 oz (small handful)
Calories	57 kcal	29 kcal
Protein	0.7 g	0.4 g
Fat	0.3 g	0.2 g
Carb	14.5 g	7.3 g
Fibre	2.4 g	1.2 g
Vitamin C	10 mg	5 mg
Vitamin E	0.6 mg	0.3 mg

Benefits

- Packed with disease-fighting antioxidants
- Boost brain power
- Help eyesight
- Fight bacteria

Nutrient powerhouses

Researchers at the US Department of Agriculture's Human Nutrition Center in Boston have found that blueberries top the list for antioxidants when compared with 40 fresh fruit and vegetables. They are packed with antioxidant vitamins C and E, but their main health benefits come from anthocyanins, the pigment that makes the berries blue. Antioxidants destroy harmful free radicals that damage cells and increase the risk of disease, so blueberries can play an important part in keeping us healthy.

Be berry wise

Blueberries are the perfect fruit for children who are studying hard and preparing for exams. American scientists have found that blueberries may boost memory, improve the ability to learn and even make us more inquisitive. This is possibly because anthocyanins protect the nerve cells.

Beat bacteria

Like cranberries, blueberries may help prevent urinary tract infections (UTIs), which affect around 3 per cent of children and are common in kids who delay trips to the bathroom. Researchers from New Jersey believe proanthocyanidins in blueberries prevent *E.coli*, the bacteria responsible for most UTIs, from attaching to the cells that line the walls of the urinary tract, causing infection.

Bright eyes

Blueberries are a great choice for teenagers who spend hours in front of a computer screen or burn the midnight oil before exams. Studies have found that anthocyanins in blueberries help to improve eyesight and ease eye fatigue.

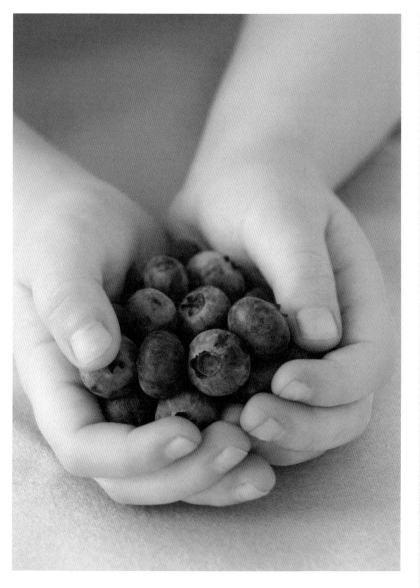

Looking forward

Getting kids into the berry habit may help to protect them from cancers and heart disease in later life. Research from the University of Mississippi has found that blueberries may reduce harmful cholesterol levels as effectively as prescribed drugs, but without any of the nasty side-effects. And it's not just thanks to their disease-fighting antioxidants, either; blueberries are also rich in pectin, a soluble fibre that helps to lower cholesterol. Laboratory research shows that blueberries may help to prevent Alzheimer's disease and even reverse short-term memory loss in elderly people, although more research is needed to confirm this.

Won't eat...
A handful of blueberries

Might eat...
A blueberry smoothie

Will eat...
A homemade blueberry muffin

Three ways
to get your kids to eat more blueberries

1 Top breakfast cereal or porridge with blueberries.

2 Mix blueberries with yogurt and a drizzle of honey for a perfect dessert.

3 Fill homemade pancakes with sliced banana, blueberries and a sprinkling of sugar, and serve with a scoop of ice cream.

Why not try...

Orange and blueberry muffins (see page 64)
Nutritional facts per muffin
229 kcal, 8.6 g fat (of which 4.8 g saturates), 16.8 g sugars, 0.3 g salt

Blueberry and lemon pancakes (see page 64)
Nutritional facts per pancake
209 kcal, 3.7 g fat (of which 1.1 g saturates), 16.4 g sugars, 0.7 g salt

Orange and blueberry muffins

● Preparation time **15 mins** ● Cooking time **20–25 mins** ● Makes **12**

50 g (2 oz) **wholemeal flour**
250 g (8 oz) **plain flour**
160 g (5½ oz) **golden caster
  sugar**
1 tsp **baking powder**
2 tsp **finely grated
  orange rind**
juice of ½ **orange**
250 ml (8 fl oz) **buttermilk**
100 g (3½ oz) **unsalted
  butter, melted**
2 **large eggs, lightly beaten**
200 g (7 oz) **blueberries**

1 Line a deep, 12-hole muffin tin with paper cases. Put the flours, sugar and baking powder in a bowl and mix well.

2 Put the orange rind and juice, buttermilk, melted butter and eggs in another bowl and stir to mix. Add the flour mixture and stir gently to combine. Take care that you do not overmix the batter.

3 Fold in the blueberries and carefully spoon the mixture into the muffin cases. Bake in a preheated oven, 190°C (375°F), Gas Mark 5, for 20–25 minutes or until lightly golden. Remove from the oven and serve warm.

Blueberry and lemon pancakes

● Preparation time **15 mins, plus chilling** ● Cooking time **about 20 mins** ● Serves **4**

125 g (4 oz) **self-raising flour**
1 tbsp **finely grated
  lemon rind**
1 tsp **baking powder**
1 tbsp **golden caster sugar**
1 **large egg, lightly beaten**
1 tbsp **orange juice**
150 ml (¼ pint) **semi-
  skimmed milk**
150 g (5 oz) **blueberries**
sunflower oil, to grease
4 tbsp **clear honey, to serve**

1 Mix together the flour, lemon rind, baking powder and sugar in a bowl.

2 In a separate bowl whisk together the egg, orange juice and milk. Pour this mixture into the dry ingredients and stir well to mix. Stir in the blueberries, cover and chill for 30 minutes.

3 Lightly grease a large, nonstick frying pan. Working in batches, drop spoonfuls of the batter, spaced well apart, into the frying pan. Cook for 2–3 minutes until bubbles appear on the surface of each pancake and the underside is lightly golden. Flip them over and cook for a further 1–2 minutes. Remove and keep warm while you cook the remaining pancakes. Serve warm, drizzled with honey.

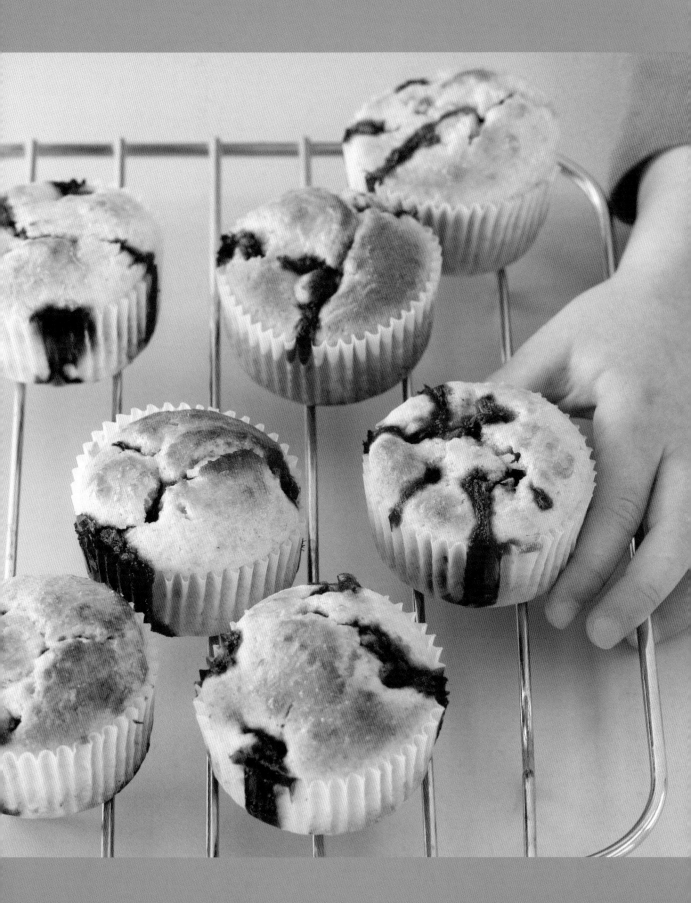

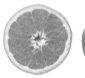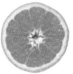

Oranges

What's in them?
Oranges

Nutrient	100 g (3½ oz)	Medium orange
Calories	37 kcal	59 kcal
Protein	1.1 g	1.8 g
Fat	0.1 g	0.2 g
Carb	8.5 g	13.6 g
Fibre	1.7 g	2.7 g
Folate	31 mcg	50 mcg
Vitamin C	54 mg	86 mg
Potassium	150 mg	240 mg

Benefits
- Heal wounds
- Boost immunity
- Healthy lung function
- Ease allergies

Encourage your kids to eat oranges; the nutrients they contain will help keep them fighting fit and give them a real zest for life.

The big squeeze
Oranges are packed with vitamin C, a nutrient that does everything from healing wounds, fighting infections and easing allergies to preventing heart disease, combating cancer and averting arthritis. But it's not just their vitamin C content that earns oranges their superfood status; they also contain fibre, potassium and folate, and a number of disease-fighting antioxidants, making them the perfect choice for your little ones.

Healing fruit
Oranges are a great food for children who constantly cut, scratch or bruise themselves as a result of falling down while playing. Vitamin C helps to strengthen capillaries (the tiniest blood vessels) and cell walls, and makes collagen. In this way, vitamin C helps to promote healing, prevent bruising and keeps tendons, ligaments and gums healthy.

Fight infection
Oranges are perfect for children susceptible to colds and bugs such as recurrent ear infections, since vitamin C is vital for a healthy immune system. Several studies show that good intakes of vitamin C ease the symptoms of a cold and speed up recovery, although it's unlikely to actually prevents colds.

Healthy lungs
Oranges are a good choice for children who suffer with chest infections or asthma. Low intakes of vitamin C are linked to respiratory infections and other lung problems, including lung cancer and asthma. In particular, a study of 6–7-year-old asthmatics found that citrus fruits helped to protect against wheezing and shortness of breath. While vitamin C almost

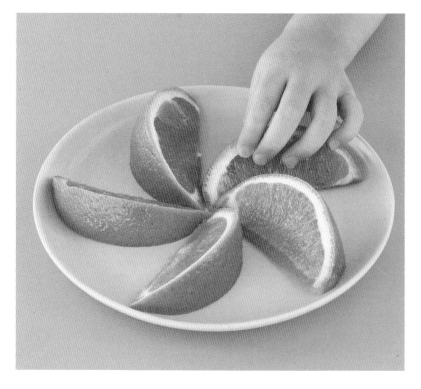

certainly has a role, oranges also contain beta-cryptoxanthin, an antioxidant that helps keep the lungs healthy (see Peppers).

Ease allergies

Good intakes of vitamin C may help to ease the symptoms associated with allergies such as hay fever or eczema. Vitamin C is a natural antihistamine that helps to control allergies by blocking inflammatory substances produced in response to allergens such as pollen and pet dander.

Give iron a boost

It is a good idea to encourage your children to drink orange juice with cereal or finish meals with an orange, especially if they are vegetarian. Vitamin C helps the body absorb the iron in vegetable foods such as cereals, green vegetables, nuts, seeds and pulses.

Looking forward

A review of 48 studies shows that diets high in citrus fruits protect against many diseases including heart disease, certain cancers, arthritis, cataracts, Alzheimer's disease, diabetes, gallstones, gum disease and Crohn's disease.

Won't eat...
A whole orange

Might eat...
Peeled orange segments

Will eat...
A glass of orange juice

Three ways
to get your kids to eat more oranges

1 Add oranges or canned mandarin segments (canned in their own juice) to fruit salad or fruit jelly.

2 Serve orange juice for breakfast or mix with sparkling water for a healthier fizzy drink.

3 Make fruit kebabs, including orange segments, and serve with a chocolate dip.

Why not try...

Orange and cranberry jelly pots (see page 68)
Nutritional facts per pot
179 kcal, 0.1 g fat (of which 0 g saturates), 18.3 g sugars, 0.1 g salt

Orange, blackberry and pineapple salad (see page 68)
Nutritional facts per portion
92 kcal, 0.4 g fat (of which 0 g saturates), 21 g sugars, 0 g salt

Orange and cranberry jelly pots

● Preparation time **15 mins, plus soaking & chilling** ● Cooking time **about 5 mins** ● Makes **4**

15 g (½ oz) **fine leaf gelatine**
600 ml (1 pint) **cranberry juice**
2 tbsp **clear honey**
2 large **oranges, peeled and cut into segments (discard the seeds and membrane), plus extra segments, to garnish**

1 Soak the gelatine in a bowl with a little cold water for 5 minutes until softened.

2 Meanwhile, place the cranberry juice and honey in a small saucepan and bring to the boil. Remove from the heat.

3 Remove the gelatine from the bowl and squeeze out any excess water. Add to the hot cranberry mixture and stir to dissolve and mix well. Allow to cool.

4 Meanwhile, line 4 dessert glasses or bowls with the orange segments. Pour over the cranberry mixture and chill in the refrigerator for 3–4 hours or until set. Serve with a spoonful of custard on top of each jelly if liked.

Orange, blackberry and pineapple salad

● Preparation time **10 mins, plus chilling** ● Serves **4**

3 **large oranges**
200 g (7 oz) **blackberries**
200 g (7 oz) **fresh pineapple, cut into bite-sized cubes**
1 tbsp **finely chopped mint leaves, to scatter (optional)**

1 Use a sharp, serrated knife to cut away the peel and pith of the oranges, saving any juices. Cut each orange into segments and remove any seeds.

2 Place the segments in a bowl with the blackberries and pineapple and stir in the mint (if used).

3 Pour over any of the saved orange juice and toss to mix well. Chill until ready to serve.

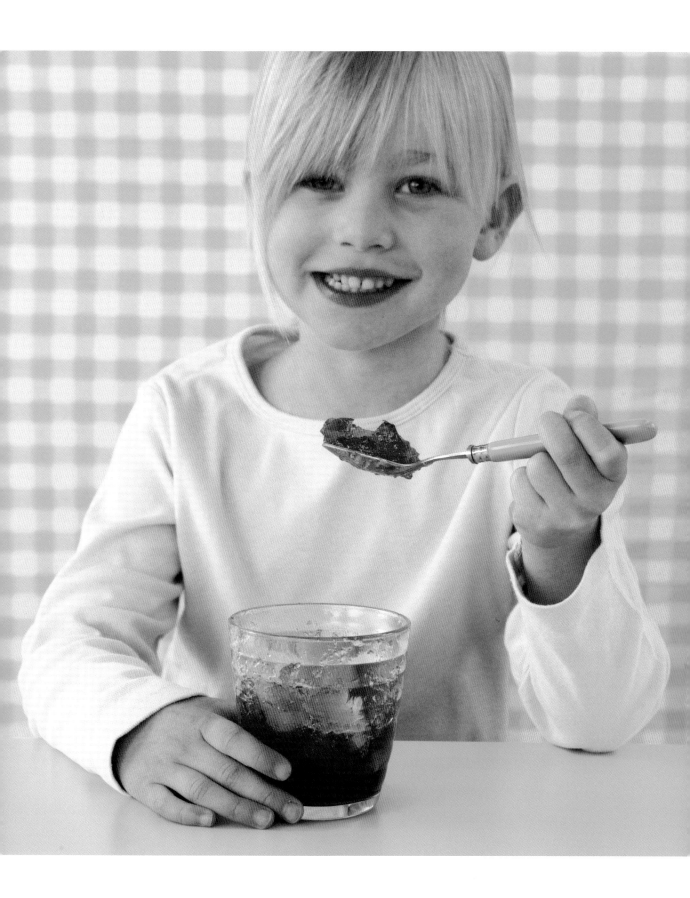

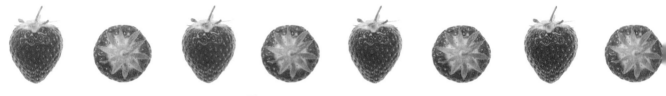

Strawberries

An apple a day may keep the doctor away, but a bowl full of strawberries may do an even better job, thanks to their unique combination of nutrients.

What's in them?
Strawberries

Nutrients	100 g 3½ oz	Per 5 straw-berries
Calories	27 kcal	16 kcal
Protein	0.8 g	0.5 g
Fat	0.1 g	0.1 g
Carb	6 g	4 g
Fibre	1.1 g	0.7 g
Folate	20 mcg	12 mcg
Vitamin C	77 mg	46 mg
Potassium	160 mg	96 mg

Benefits
- Natural painkiller
- Ease allergies
- Improve eyesight
- Boost memory

Berry good for you
Strawberries are one of the few sweet treats that also have numerous health benefits. These little red fruits keep the heart healthy, reduce the risk of cancer, improve vision, prevent allergies and even ease pain, making them a great choice for children. Strawberries are packed with fibre and vitamin C and contain smaller amounts of folate and potassium, but they earn their rank as a miracle food because of their antioxidant nutrients.

Diet divas
Children who eat strawberries generally have better diets overall. A study of 1–19-year-olds found those who ate strawberries had higher intakes of fibre, vitamin C and carotenes, and lower body-mass indexes, weights and waist circumferences, suggesting they were less likely to be overweight. Research also shows that adults who eat strawberries tend to have healthier diets and know more about healthy eating – a good enough reason to get children into the strawberry-eating habit early on.

Natural pain relief
Giving children strawberries when they are in pain may be a tasty alternative to traditional painkillers. Strawberries contain naturally occurring plant chemicals called phenols, which work in a similar way to painkillers like aspirin and ibuprofen by blocking the activity of an enzyme that contributes to inflammation.

Smarter children
Snacking on strawberries when studying may help children perform better in tests and exams. Like blueberries, strawberries contain anthocyanin, an antioxidant that provides their red colour and may improve short-term memory (see Blueberries).

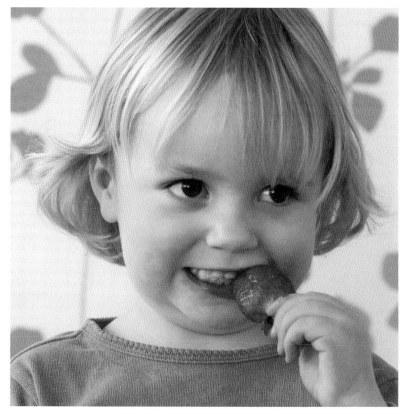

Prevent allergies

Strawberries contain an antioxidant quercetin that inhibits the release of histamine, a natural substance produced by the body when there is an allergy. Histamine causes many of the typical symptoms seen with allergy, such as itchy eyes, nose and skin, rashes, hives, wheezing and headaches. While anti-histamine medication reduces these symptoms, giving children strawberries may also help – providing they are not allergic to them.

Better vision

Like blueberries, anthocyanins in strawberries have been linked to better eyesight and so may help children in class and with studying that involves a lot of reading or computer work (see Blueberries).

Looking forward

The antioxidants in strawberries have been shown to reduce the risk of heart disease, stroke, certain cancers and even inhibit *Helicobacter pylori,* a bacterium that causes stomach ulcers.

Won't eat...
Whole strawberries

Might eat...
Sliced strawberries with vanilla ice cream

Will eat...
Strawberry milkshake

Three ways
to get your kids to eat more strawberries

1 Make a fruit jelly using reduced-sugar jelly crystals and sliced, fresh strawberries.

2 Make strawberry and yogurt smoothies or simply mix chopped strawberries into strawberry yogurt.

3 Make your own strawberry scones, muffins or bread.

Why not try...

Strawberry smoothies
(see page 72)
Nutritional facts per portion
107 kcal, 1.5 g fat (of which 0.9 g saturates), 18.7 g sugars, 0.1 g salt

Marbled strawberry ice lollies (see page 72)
Nutritional facts per lolly
45 kcal, 0.4 g fat (of which 0.3 g saturates), 8.6 g sugars, 0.1 g salt

Strawberry smoothies

● Preparation time **10 mins, plus chilling** ● Serves **4**

300 g (10 oz) **strawberries, hulled and roughly chopped**
1 **ripe banana**
200 g (7 oz) **low-fat yogurt**
200 ml (7 fl oz) **semi-skimmed milk**
2 tsp **clear honey**

1 Put half of the strawberries in a juicer or food processor. Peel and chop the banana and add to the strawberries together with the yogurt, milk and honey.

2 Process until thick and smooth, adding a little more milk if you want a thinner consistency. Add the remaining strawberries and process for a few seconds until the smoothie has a marbled effect. Serve chilled.

Marbled strawberry ice lollies

● Preparation time **10 mins, plus freezing** ● Makes **6**

300 g (10 oz) **ripe strawberries, hulled and roughly chopped**
2 tsp **golden caster sugar**
200 ml (7 fl oz) **vanilla-flavoured low-fat yogurt**

1 Put the strawberries and sugar in a food processor or blender and process until smooth. Transfer to a bowl.

2 Stir the yogurt until smooth and then gently spoon into the strawberry purée. Stir gently to create a marbled effect.

3 Spoon the marbled mixture into 6 ice-lolly moulds and freeze for 4–6 hours or until frozen. To serve, dip the moulds in hot water for a few seconds and unmould.

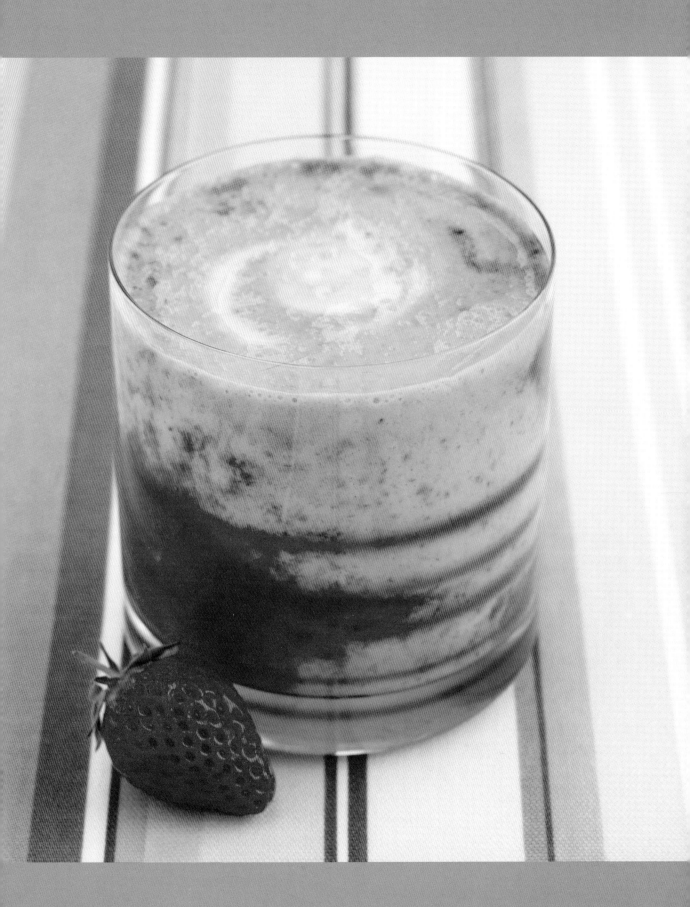

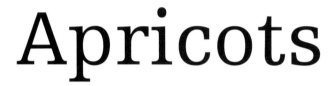

Apricots

The sweet taste of apricots will be a winner with your young ones when you add them to cereals, stews or smoothies.

What's in them?
Dried apricots

Nutrient	100 g (3½ oz)	1 dried apricot
Calories	158 kcal	13 kcal
Protein	4 g	0.3 g
Fat	0.6 g	0 g
Carb	36.5 g	2.9 g
Fibre	6.3 g	0.5 g
Potassium	1,380 mg	110 mg
Iron	3.4 mg	0.3 mg
Copper	0.4 mg	0.03 mg

Benefits
- A sweet treat
- Boost energy
- Lower blood pressure

The versatile fruit

Apricots might be small but they pack a powerful nutritional punch with good amounts of fibre, potassium, iron and copper, and smaller quantities of calcium and beta-carotene. In particular, dried apricots are a concentrated source of nutrients, containing four times more fibre, five times more potassium and calcium, and seven times more iron than an equal weight of fresh ones. This makes dried apricots a great choice for young children with small tummies who need to get plenty of nutrients from a small amount of food. They are also versatile and can be used in sweet or savoury dishes to add taste and texture.

A sweet treat

Apricots are naturally sweet and make a great alternative to sweets and chocolate, which contain few nutrients. Babies are born with a preference for sweet foods – breast milk is much sweeter than cows' milk, for example – and this continues into childhood, explaining why most children love confectionery, biscuits and sugary drinks. Dried apricots give children a sweet treat, while topping up fibre, vitamins and minerals.

Under pressure

Apricots can help boost potassium, a mineral that keeps the kidneys, heart, nerves and muscles functioning normally. Unfortunately, many teenagers fail to get enough potassium. According to the last National Diet and Nutrition Survey of Young People conducted in the UK, one in seven boys and one in three girls aged 15–18 years have potassium levels below the minimum amount recommended for good health. This is worrying as some studies link low potassium with high blood pressure in later life.

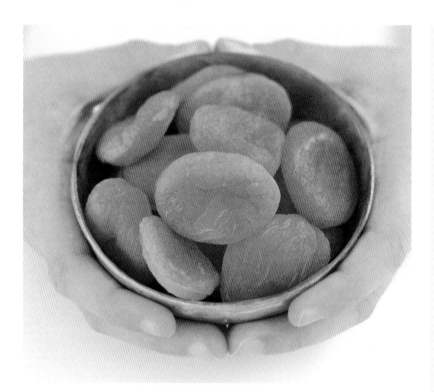

Won't eat...
Fresh apricots

Might eat...
Dried apricots

Will eat...
Ice cream with apricot purée

Three ways
to get your kids to eat more apricots

1 Add fresh or dried apricots to breakfast cereal or porridge.

2 Serve pancakes with ice cream and fresh or canned apricots for dessert.

3 Add dried apricots to chicken or pork stews, casseroles and rice dishes.

Energy providers
Dried apricots can boost energy levels in children as they are a concentrated source of calories. Plus, they help to keep nerves and muscles topped up with potassium, which helps to prevent fatigue. This is especially important in hot weather when more potassium is lost in sweat.

Easy way to five-a-day
Apricots are an easy way to get children eating one of their five daily portions of fruit and vegetables. Just three whole fresh, dried or ready-to-eat apricots count as one serving.

Get canned
Don't be afraid to buy canned apricots (in natural juice not syrup). Research from the University of Illinois shows they contain just as many nutrients as fresh apricots.

Looking forward
The potassium in apricots may help to prevent high blood pressure, while beta-carotene may protect against cancer and heart disease.

Why not try...

Apricot and yogurt breakfast pots (see page 76)
Nutritional facts per pot
182 kcal, 2.1 g fat (of which 0.3 g saturates), 25.6 g sugars, 0.1 g salt

Apricot & cherry brochettes with apple cream (see page 76)
Nutritional facts per brochette
110 kcal, 6.1 g fat (of which 1.2 g saturates), 9.7 g sugars, 0 g salt

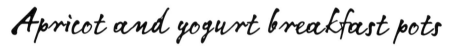

Apricot and yogurt breakfast pots

● Preparation time **15 mins** ● Cooking time **6–8 mins** ● Makes **4**

200 g (7 oz) **ready-to-eat dried apricots**
1 **stick of cinnamon**
200 g (7 oz) **low-fat Greek yogurt**
4 tbsp **rolled oats**
1–2 tbsp **clear honey, to drizzle**

1 Roughly chop the apricots and place them in a small saucepan with the cinnamon stick. Just cover with water and bring to the boil. Reduce the heat and allow to simmer gently for 6–8 minutes.

2 Remove the cinnamon stick and discard. Transfer the apricot mixture to a food processor or blender and process until smooth, adding a little more water if the mixture is too thick.

3 Spoon the apricot compote into the base of 4 individual pots or ramekins. Top with the yogurt, sprinkle over the oats and serve, drizzled with honey.

Apricot & cherry brochettes with apple cream

● Preparation time **20 mins, plus chilling** ● Makes **8**

100 g (3½ oz) **unsalted cashew nuts**
125 ml (4 fl oz) **organic apple juice**
16 **ripe apricots, halved and stoned**
32 **ripe, sweet cherries, pitted**
icing sugar, to dust
mint leaves, to garnish (optional)

1 Make the apple cream. Put the cashew nuts in a food processor or blender and process to a fine mixture. Continue to blend until the nuts start to clump together. Add the apple juice, a little at a time, blending after each addition, until all the juice is used up and the mixture is pale and creamy. Transfer to a small bowl, cover and chill for 2–3 hours.

2 Cut the apricot halves into wedges and thread apricot pieces and cherries alternately on to 8 wooden or presoaked bamboo skewers.

3 Arrange the skewers on a serving platter with the bowl of apple cream as a dip. Dust with icing sugar and garnish with mint leaves (if used).

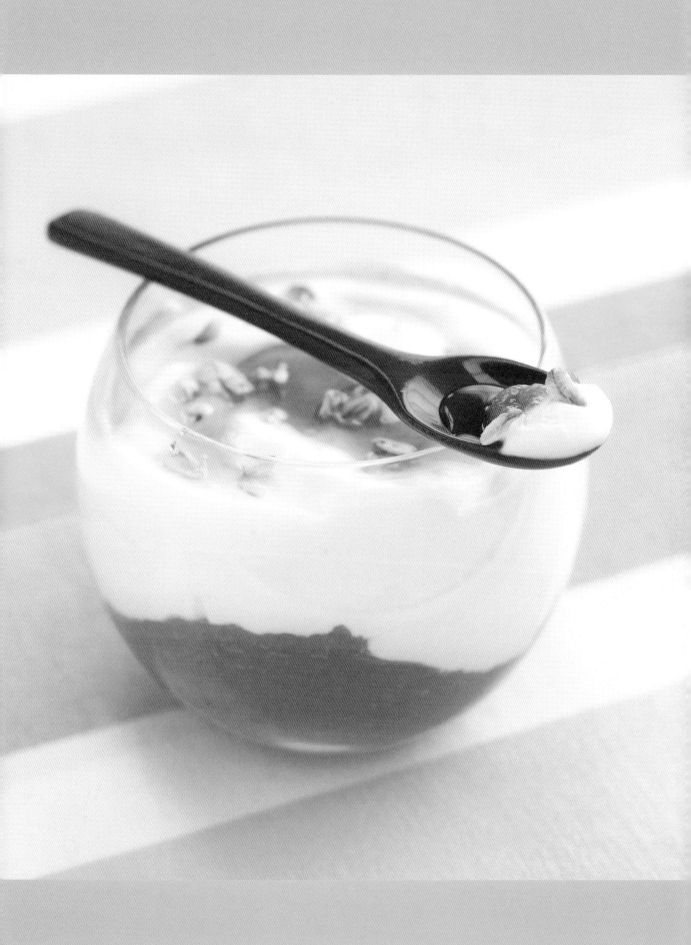

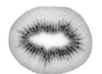

Kiwifruit

What's in them?
Kiwifruit

Nutrient	100 g (3½ oz)	1 kiwifruit
Calories	49 kcal	29 kcal
Protein	1.1 g	0.7 g
Fat	0.5 g	0.3 g
Carb	10.6 g	6.4 g
Fibre	1.9 g	1.1 g
Vitamin C	59 mg	35 mg
Vitamin E	1.5 mg	0.9 mg
Potassium	290 mg	174 mg

Benefits
- Healthy breathing
- Repairs cells
- Keeps eyes healthy

Eaten like a boiled egg with a spoon, this is one little fruit guaranteed to be a hit with children's tastebuds and tummies.

Fruity facts
It's only when you cut open this brown, furry fruit that the true health benefits are released. Kiwifruits, sometimes called Chinese gooseberries, are actually berries and their edible seeds provide many nutrients. According to a study published in the *Journal of the American College of Nutrition*, out of 27 fruits, kiwifruits are the most nutrient-dense of all, above apples, bananas and peaches. In particular, they contain fibre and potassium and are rich in vitamins C and E. Just one kiwifruit a day provides all the vitamin C needed by children under the age of 15. This makes them a great choice for kids who won't eat citrus fruits.

Ease the wheeze
For children who suffer with breathing difficulties, a kiwifruit a day might just keep the doctor away. In a study of Italian children aged 6–7 years, almost half of those who ate the most citrus fruit and kiwifruit were less likely to wheeze compared with those children who ate the least. Furthermore, shortness of breath was reduced by a third, while coughing at night, chronic coughing and a runny nose were reduced by around a quarter. Asthmatic children benefited most. The vitamin C in kiwifruit is likely to be partly responsible for this beneficial effect as this nutrient helps to keep the lungs healthy (see Oranges).

Repairing cells
Research from the Rowett Research Institute in Scotland reveals that kiwifruit can help to protect against, and even fix, cell damage that can cause cancer. Just one kiwifruit a day was found to repair damage to DNA – the part of the cell that carries genetic information – with higher intakes leading to even greater repair.

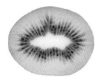 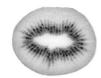 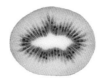 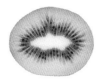

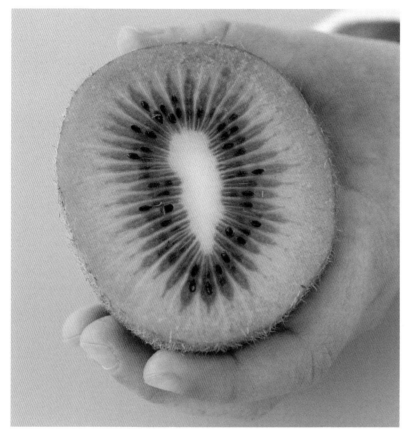

Won't eat...
A kiwifruit

Might eat...
Kiwifruit in jelly

Will eat...
Pancakes filled with
kiwifruit and ice cream

Three ways
**to get your kids to eat
more kiwifruit**

1 Fill meringue nests
with chopped kiwifruit
and strawberries and top
with a little reduced-fat
aerosol cream.

2 Blend kiwifruit with
other favourite fruits
to make a smoothie.

3 Make kebabs using
pieces of kiwi and other
favourite fruit.

Why not try...

Kiwifruit and blueberry pavlovas (see page 80)
Nutritional facts per pavlova
**69 kcal, 0.4 g fat (of which 0.2 g
saturates), 15.8 g sugars, 0.1 g salt**

Kiwifruit and raspberry mousse (see page 80)
Nutritional facts per portion
**184 kcal, 7.3 g fat (of which 4.7 g
saturates), 21 g sugars, 0.7 g salt**

The green party

Kiwifruit are a great choice for kids who won't eat greens such
as sprouts, cabbage and broccoli, since the fruit contains an
antioxidant called lutein, which is typically found in green
vegetables (see Broccoli). As well as helping to reduce heart
disease and cancer, this nutrient is important for healthy vision.

A healthy heart

Getting kids into the habit of eating kiwifruit may help to ensure
their hearts stay healthy in later life. In one study, people who
ate two or three kiwifruit every day for a month saw their
potential for forming blood clots drop by 18 per cent and a type
of blood fat called triglycerides drop by 15 per cent.

Looking forward

Thanks to their vitamin C and other antioxidant content,
kiwifruits have the potential to protect against many diseases
including heart disease, cancer, eye problems and arthritis.

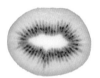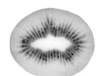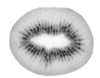

Kiwifruit and blueberry pavlovas

● Preparation time **20 mins** ● Cooking time **1¾–2 hours** ● Makes **10**

Meringues
2 **egg whites (at room temperature)**
100 g (3½ oz) **golden caster sugar**
Topping
4 **kiwifruit**
100 g (3½ oz) **blueberries**
200 ml (7 fl oz) **vanilla- or fruit-flavoured low-fat yogurt**

1 Grease and line 2 baking sheets. Place the egg whites in a large, grease-free mixing bowl and use a hand-held electric whisk to beat them until they are fairly stiff. (You should be able to turn the bowl upside down without any spillage.) Continue whisking, adding the sugar 1 tablespoon at a time, until the mixture is stiff and glossy.

2 Place 10 tablespoons of the mixture, spaced well apart, on the prepared trays, making a small hollow in the centre of each one for the filling. Bake in a preheated oven, 120°C (250°F), Gas Mark ½, for 1¾–2 hours.

3 Meanwhile, peel the kiwifruit and chop the flesh into 1 cm (½ inch) pieces. Mix with the blueberries.

4 Place the meringues in serving dishes. Spoon some yogurt into the centre of each meringue and top with the fruit. Eat immediately.

Kiwifruit and raspberry mousse

● Preparation time **15 mins, plus chilling** ● Serves **4**

250 g (8 oz) **low-fat soft cheese**
100 ml (3½ fl oz) **fromage frais**
50 g (2 oz) **icing sugar**
150 g (5 oz) **fresh raspberries**
2 **large kiwifruit, peeled and cut into 1 cm (½ inch) dice**

1 Place the cream cheese and fromage frais in a bowl and beat with a wooden spoon until smooth. Stir in the icing sugar and mix well.

2 Add the raspberries and stir until they are marbled through and just beginning to release their juices into the cheese mixture.

3 Fold in the kiwifruit (reserving some pieces for the garnish) until well mixed. Spoon this mixture into chilled dessert bowls or glasses and top with the reserved kiwifruit. Serve chilled.

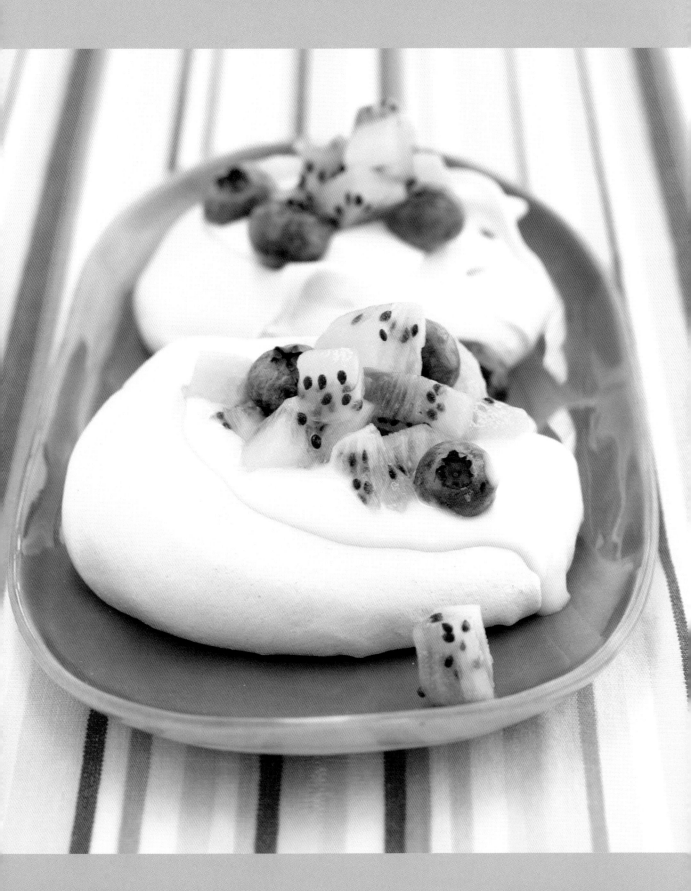

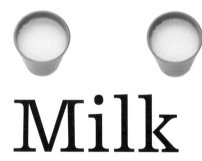

Milk

What's in it?
Semi-skimmed milk

Nutrient	100 g (3½ oz)	200 ml glass
Calories	46 kcal	92 kcal
Protein	3.5 g	7 g
Fat	1.7 g	3.4 g
Carb	4.7 g	9.4 g
Vitamin A	21 mcg	42 mcg
Vitamin B2	0.2 mg	0.4 mg
Vitamin B12	0.9 mcg	1.8 mcg
Calcium	120 mg	240 mg
Phosphorus	94 mg	188 mg
Iodine	30 mcg	60 mcg

Benefits
- Builds strong bones
- Prevents osteoporosis
- Healthy teeth
- Helps with weight control

With its unique combination of essential nutrients, milk is one food all parents should bone up on, no matter how old their children are.

Building healthy bones

Milk is packed with vitamins A (in full-fat and semi-skimmed milk), B2 and B12, plus phosphorus and iodine. But its true superfood status comes from the bone-building calcium it contains. Children's bones grow quickly and research shows that more than 90 per cent of the calcium that individuals will ever have in their bones is already there by the age of 17, making childhood and the teenage years the crucial time for depositing calcium in the bone bank. Unfortunately, the UK's National Diet and Nutrition Survey of Young People reveals that around one in five 11–18-year-old girls and one in ten boys of the same age don't get enough calcium.

Preventing osteoporosis

While osteoporosis is not usually a problem in children and teenagers, the calcium intakes during this time are what helps to prevent this disease in later life. By middle age bones start to lose calcium faster than they store it and so gradually lose their strength. Osteoporosis, which currently affects one woman in two and one man in five over the age of 50 in the UK, occurs when the bones become so weak they fracture easily. The more calcium deposited in the bone bank during childhood and teenage years, the stronger that bone bank will be in later life – and the greater the protection against osteoporosis.

Absorbing news

The calcium in milk and yogurt is more easily absorbed and used by the body than the calcium in non-dairy foods – another good reason to encourage kids to keep the milk habit. Remember under twos should have full-fat milk and don't give skimmed milk to children under five (see Introduction).

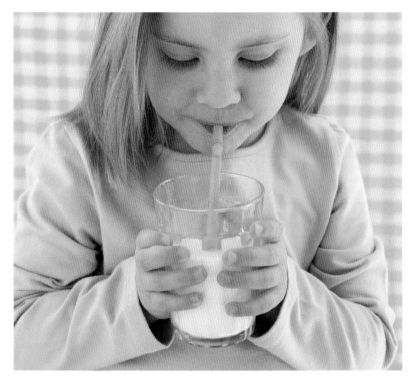

Stop teething troubles

Drinking milk helps give children strong, healthy teeth. Calcium is an essential part of dentine that is laid down in early childhood and forms the main part of the tooth beneath the enamel. Milk is also less likely to cause tooth decay than sugary fizzy drinks, squashes and fruit juices.

Fight fat

Milk may prevent obesity in children and teenagers – studies show that higher calcium intakes from dairy products are linked to less body fat in children. Plus, a study from Cornell University found that children who drank more milk and fewer sweetened drinks gained less weight over two months.

Looking forward

Research shows that good intakes of calcium from dairy products may help adults to lose fat from around their middle. Meanwhile, low-fat milk and dairy products can lower blood pressure. Milk is also one of the few foods to contain CLA (see Beef), which may help to prevent heart disease and cancer, and boost immunity.

Won't drink...
A glass of milk

Might drink...
Milk with cereal

Will eat...
Home-made banana custard

Three ways
to get your kids to drink more milk

1 Top pasta with homemade cheese sauce made using semi-skimmed milk.

2 Encourage kids to have homemade milkshakes or smoothies rather than fizzy drinks.

3 Get teenagers to make 'skinny' lattes or cappuccinos using skimmed or semi-skimmed milk rather than regular coffee with a dash of milk.

Why not try...

Cheesy cauliflower grill
(see page 84)
Nutritional facts per portion
224 kcal, 9.2 g fat (of which 5.45 g saturates, 7.9 sugars, 0.6 salt

Vanilla and orange baked custards (see page 84)
Nutritional facts per custard
165 kcal, 6.4 g fat (of which 2.3 g saturates), 21.4 g sugars, 0.2 g salt

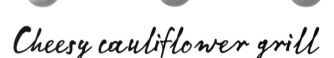

Cheesy cauliflower grill

● Preparation time **20 mins** ● Cooking time **about 15 mins** ● Serves **6**

450 g (14½ oz) **cauliflower, cut into small florets**
25 g (1 oz) **unsalted butter**
3 tbsp **plain flour**
700 ml (25 fl oz) **semi-skimmed milk, warmed**
1 tsp **dried mixed herbs**
¼ tsp **ground cinnamon**
50 g (2 oz) **Cheddar cheese, grated**
5 tbsp **fresh wholemeal breadcrumbs**
pepper

1 Steam or boil the cauliflower for 5–6 minutes or until just tender. Drain and place in a gratin or shallow ovenproof dish.

2 Put the butter in a nonstick saucepan and melt over a low heat. Add the flour and cook, stirring, for 3–4 minutes or until the mixture is lightly browned. Gradually pour in the warm milk, whisking constantly as you do so. Add the mixed herbs and cinnamon. Cook, stirring, for 6–8 minutes until the mixture is thickened and forms a smooth sauce.

3 Stir in the cheese, season with pepper and mix until smooth. Pour this mixture over the prepared cauliflower and toss to mix well. Sprinkle over the breadcrumbs and place under a medium-hot grill until the top is golden and bubbling.

Vanilla and orange baked custards

● Preparation time **20 mins** ● Cooking time **1¼ hours** ● Serves **6**

500 ml (17 fl oz) **semi-skimmed milk**
1 **vanilla pod, split in half**
100 g (3½ oz) **golden caster sugar**
2 **eggs and 3 yolks**
2 tsp **finely grated orange rind**

1 Place the milk in a saucepan with the vanilla pod and half the sugar and bring to the boil. Remove from the heat and allow the flavours to infuse.

2 In a large bowl whisk the eggs and yolks with the remaining sugar until thick and frothy.

3 Remove the vanilla pod from the milk and pour the slightly cooled liquid over the egg mixture, whisking constantly, until well blended. Stir in the orange rind.

4 Strain the custard into 6 individual ovenproof ramekins and place them in a deep roasting tin. Fill the tin with boiling water so that it comes halfway up the sides of the ramekins. Bake in a preheated oven, 180°C (350°F), Gas Mark 4, for about 1 hour or until the custards are just firm. Remove from the oven, leave to cool, then chill for 4–5 hours. Serve the custards with mixed fruit salad if liked.

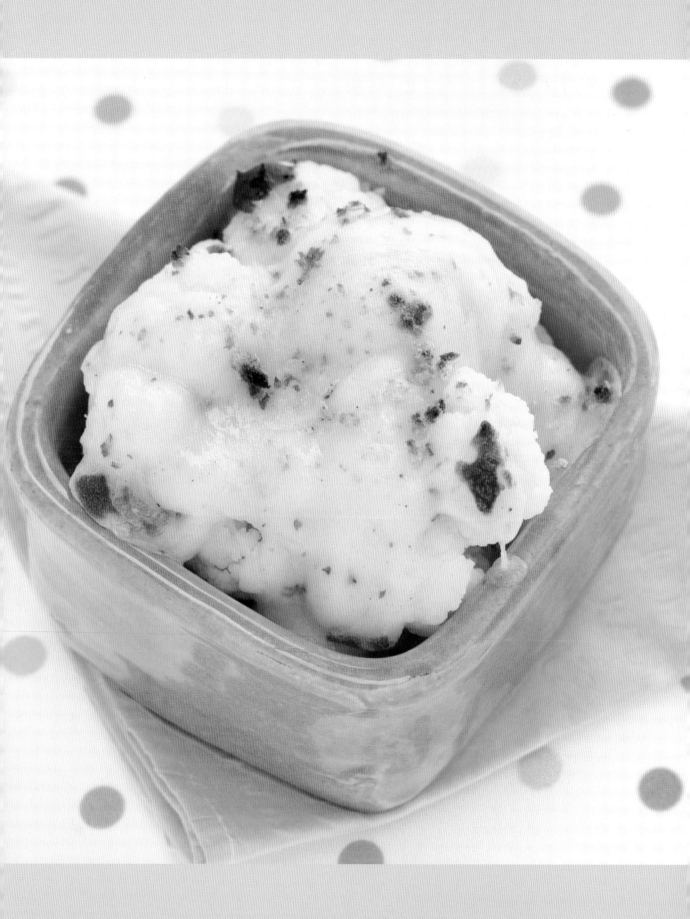

Yogurt

What's in it?
Natural low-fat yogurt

Nutrient	100 g 3½ oz	150 g/5 fl oz small pot
Calories	56 kcal	84 kcal
Protein	4.8 g	72 g
Fat	1 g	1.5 g
Carb	7.4 g	11.1 g
Vitamin B2	0.2 mg	0.3 mg
Vitamin B12	0.3 mcg	0.5 mcg
Calcium	162 mg	243 mg
Phosphorus	143 mg	215 mg
Iodine	34 mcg	51 mcg

Benefits
- **Keeps the digestive tract healthy**
- **Boosts immunity**
- **Fights thrush**
- **Prevents osteoporosis**
- **Aids weight loss**

Adding a little culture to your child's mealtimes can do everything from boosting immunity to keeping the digestive system healthy.

Yummy yogurt
Yogurt is made by adding bacteria to milk, which causes it to ferment and thicken. This means, that like milk, yogurt is packed with vitamins B2 and B12, phosphorus and iodine. Plus it's a great source of calcium and so helps to build strong bones and teeth and aids weight control. But research increasingly shows that yogurt has many other health benefits.

Treats tummy troubles
Encouraging your child to eat yogurt after a tummy upset may help to prevent further problems. This is because certain bacteria found in live yogurt may keep the digestive system healthy by increasing the levels of 'friendly' bacteria in the gut. For example, specific strains of *Lactobacillus* bacteria have been shown to reduce the severity and duration of infectious diarrhoea in toddlers and children.

Up the anti
Get your kids to eat yogurt if they are taking antibiotics as this can help to replenish levels of friendly bacteria in the digestive tract that antibiotics typically destroy.

Lactose intolerance
Some children with lactose intolerance can still tolerate yogurt without side-effects, making it easier for them to take in enough calcium for healthy bone-building. Lactose intolerance is caused by a deficiency in lactase, the enzyme that digests lactose (the main sugar in milk). It's often a temporary side effet of having a period of diarrhoea. Research shows that different bacteria in yogurt, including *Lactobacillus acidophilus* and *Bifidobacteria*, help to improve tolerance to lactose.

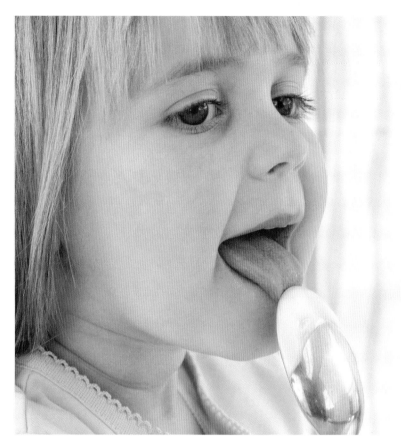

Fight infection

Certain bacteria in yogurt may help to boost immunity, preventing common childhood problems such as coughs and colds.

Eat to beat thrush

Live bacteria in yogurt may help to prevent thrush, a common yeast infection in toddlers that can occur with weakened immunity or when antibiotics disturb the balance of bacteria in the body.

Looking forward

Thanks to its calcium content, yogurt may help aid fat loss from around the midriff. Good intakes of calcium from yogurt during childhood can also help to protect against osteoporosis. Yogurt may help keep the digestive system healthy by boosting levels of friendly bacteria in the gut; certain live cultures in yogurt may even help to destroy *Helicobater pylori,* the bacterium responsible for stomach ulcers.

Won't eat...
A pot of yogurt

Might eat...
A yogurt and fruit smoothie

Will eat...
Meatballs in pitta bread drizzled with tzatziki

Three ways
to get your kids to eat more yogurt

1 Swirl puréed fruit and a drizzle of honey in natural yogurt.

2 For a tasty after-school snack, make a dip by combining yogurt, grated cucumber, mint and lemon juice and serve with warm pitta bread.

3 Top breakfast cereals with yogurt as a change from milk.

Why not try...

Mango and yogurt brûlées (see page 88)
Nutritional facts per portion
171 kcal, 1.4 g fat (of which 0.8 g saturates), 36.1 g sugars, 0.2 g salt

Moussaka (see page 88)
Nutritional facts per portion
230 kcal, 9.9 g fat (of which 5.8 g saturates), 10.4 g sugars, 0.6 g salt

Mango and yogurt brûlées

● Preparation time **10 mins, plus standing** ● Makes **4**

1 **large, ripe mango**
600 ml (1 pint) **vanilla-flavoured low-fat yogurt**
4 tsp **soft brown sugar**

1 Peel the mango and cut the flesh from the stone. Roughly chop the flesh and divide it among 4 individual ramekins or dessert bowls. Spoon over the yogurt.

2 Lightly sprinkle the sugar over the top of the yogurt and leave for 10–12 minutes to soften. Swirl the sugar through the yogurt and serve immediately.

Moussaka

● Preparation time **30 mins** ● Cooking time **55–70 minutes** ● Serves **6**

2 **large potatoes**
3 **aubergines**
2 **garlic cloves, crushed**
3 tbsp **finely chopped fresh coriander leaves**
8 **spring onions, finely chopped**
4 **ripe tomatoes, finely chopped**
2 tbsp **tomato purée**
1 tsp **ground cinnamon**
350 ml (12 fl oz) **natural low-fat yogurt**
75 g (3 oz) **Gruyère or Parmesan cheese, grated**
grated nutmeg
pepper

1 Parboil the potatoes for 10–12 minutes, drain and slice them. Set aside.

2 Meanwhile, put the whole aubergines on a baking tray and cook in a preheated oven, 220°C (425°F), Gas Mark 7, for 25–30 minutes or until softened. Remove from the oven and, when they are cool enough to handle, scoop out the flesh and discard the skins. Place the flesh in a bowl, mash it with the garlic and coriander and stir to mix well. Set aside. Reduce the oven temperature to 180°C (350°F), Gas Mark 4.

3 Thoroughly mix the spring onions with the tomatoes, tomato purée and cinnamon.

4 Assemble the moussaka. Put a layer of sliced potatoes in the base of a deep, medium-sized ovenproof dish. Spread a layer of the aubergine mixture over. Top with the tomato mixture. Continue to layer, finishing with the potatoes or aubergine.

5 Whisk the yogurt until smooth and stir in the cheese. Season with nutmeg and pepper and pour this mixture over the top to cover. Bake for 30–40 minutes or until the top is golden and bubbling.

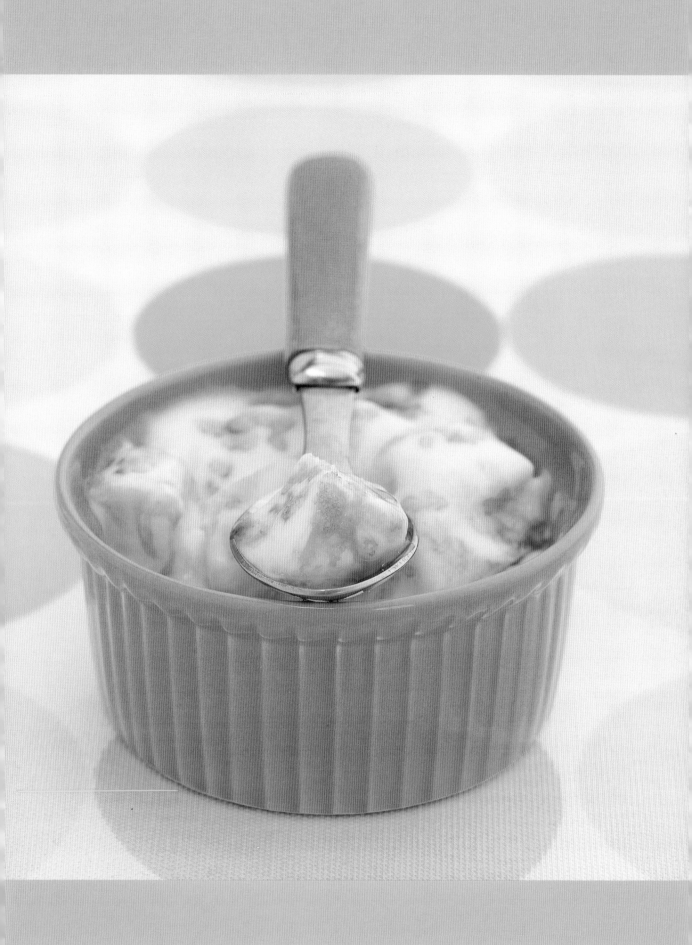

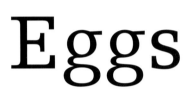

Eggs

What's in them?
Boiled eggs

Nutrient	100 g (3½ oz)	1 egg
Calories	147 kcal	87 kcal
Protein	12.5 g	7.4 g
Fat	10.8 g	6.4 g
Carb	0 g	0 g
Vitamin A	190 mcg	112 mcg
Vitamin B2	0.4 mg	0.2 mg
Vitamin B3	3.8 mg	2.2 mg
Vitamin B12	1.1 mcg	0.6 mcg
Vitamin D	1.8 mcg	1.1 mcg
Vitamin E	1.1 mg	0.6 mg
Phosphorus	200 mg	118 mg
Iron	1.9 mg	1.1 mg
Zinc	1.3 mg	0.8 mg
Selenium	11 mcg	6.5 mcg

Benefits
- Good for behaviour
- Boosts memory
- Healthy bones
- Beauty booster

Eggs have come in for some criticism in the past, but new research shows that eggs nourish children's brains and may even improve their behaviour.

Egg-cellent news

You don't need to restrict the number of eggs your children eat. In the past, health experts recommended limiting egg consumption because of their high cholesterol content. However, more than 200 studies show that the cholesterol in food, including eggs, has less effect on the blood cholesterol levels than the amount of saturates we eat. As a result, the Food Standards Agency doesn't put a limit on egg consumption. This is great news as eggs are packed with nutrients that help keep little ones healthy, including vitamins A, D and E, B vitamins, phosphorus, zinc, selenium, iron and chromium.

Good eggs

The iron, zinc, B vitamins and protein in eggs may help prevent behaviour problems in children. According to a study in the *American Journal of Psychiatry*, three-year-olds who had diets deficient in these nutrients had lower IQs and were 41 per cent more likely to be aggressive by the age of eight. By 17, they were twice as likely to be violent and exhibit antisocial behaviour. The researchers believe these nutrients affect behaviour because they are needed for a healthy nervous system, which in turn is important for mental and emotional health.

Memory tests

Eating eggs may improve children's memories as they contain choline, a nutrient needed for the development of the brain's learning and memory centres. Animal studies show that offspring who don't get enough choline in the womb have poorer memories, while those who receive choline supplements and have a greater learning capacity. Research is needed to confirm these findings and to discover whether giving young children foods rich in choline benefits memory.

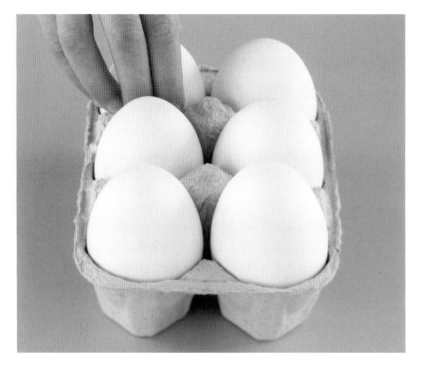

Bone up

Eggs contain bone-strengthening phosphorus and are rich in vitamin D, which absorbs calcium in the intestine, helping to build healthy bones. A lack of vitamin D causes rickets, characterized by deformed, bow-shaped legs.

Beauty boost

Eggs are a great choice for image-conscious teenage girls as they contain biotin, a vitamin that keeps nails and hair healthy. Eggs also contain good amounts of 'beauty mineral' sulphur (see Cod).

Control blood sugar

Eggs are rich in chromium, a trace mineral that may help to prevent Type 2 diabetes by enabling the body to use insulin more efficiently. Chromium can also help to stop blood-sugar levels dropping so low that children get headaches or feel irritable.

Looking forward

New research shows eggs may help to prevent heart disease by improving blood cholesterol profiles and stopping clots. Eating eggs for breakfast may also help obese women lose weight by cutting calorie intake for the rest of the day.

Won't eat...
A boiled egg

Might eat...
An egg mayonnaise sandwich

Will eat...
A cheese omelette

Three ways
to get your kids to eat more eggs

1 Make egg custard for dessert.

2 Add a hard-boiled egg to packed lunches.

3 Fill sandwiches or baked potatoes with eggs mixed with reduced-fat mayonnaise and cress.

Why not try...

Mexican-style baked eggs
(see page 92)
Nutritional facts per portion
103 kcal, 6.5 g fat (of which 1.6 g saturates), 4.8 g sugars, 0.2 g salt

Vegetable egg rolls
(see page 92)
Nutritional facts per roll
169 kcal, 12.6 g fat (of which 2.6 g saturates), 2.2 g sugars, 1 g salt

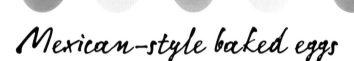

Mexican-style baked eggs

- Preparation time **20 mins** ● Cooking time **70–82 mins** ● Serves **6**

1 tbsp **olive oil**
1 **small onion, finely chopped**
2 **garlic cloves, finely chopped**
1 **red pepper, cored,
  deseeded and finely
  chopped**
2 x 400 g (13 oz) **cans
  chopped tomatoes**
1 tsp **golden caster sugar**
1 tsp **ground cumin**
pinch of **dried chilli flakes
  (optional)**
6 **eggs**

1 Heat the oil in a large, nonstick frying pan. Add the onion, garlic and red pepper, stir and cook over a medium heat for 10–12 minutes.

2 Add the tomatoes, sugar, cumin and chilli (if used) and bring to the boil. Reduce the heat and cook for 40–45 minutes, stirring occasionally or until the mixture is thick.

3 Transfer the tomato mixture to a large, shallow ovenproof dish. Level the mixture and make 6 shallow, evenly spaced hollows in the surface of the mixture with the back of a spoon. Carefully break an egg into each hollow. Bake in a preheated oven, 200°C (400°F), Gas Mark 6, for 20–25 minutes or until the eggs have set.

Vegetable egg rolls

- Preparation time **20 mins** ● Cooking time **about 15 mins** ● Makes **4**

Filling:
1 tbsp **sunflower oil**
4 **spring onions, finely
  shredded**
1 **garlic clove, crushed**
¼ **red pepper, cored,
  deseeded and finely diced**
½ **courgette, fincly diced**
2–3 tbsp **bean sprouts**
1 tbsp **reduced-salt, dark
  soy sauce**
2 tsp **cornflour**
1 tsp **sesame oil**
1 tbsp **rice wine vinegar**
4 **eggs**
2 tbsp **fresh coriander
  leaves, finely chopped**
sunflower oil, for greasing

1 Make the filling. Heat the oil in a large, nonstick frying pan or wok. Add the spring onions and garlic, stir, then turn the heat to high and add the red pepper, courgette and bean sprouts. Stir-fry for 3–4 minutes until slightly softened.

2 In a small bowl mix the soy sauce, cornflower, sesame oil and rice wine vinegar with 1 tablespoon cold water and add to the vegetable mixture. Stir thoroughly to mix and stir-fry for 2–3 minutes. Remove from the heat, cover and keep warm.

3 Beat the eggs in a measuring jug with 2 tablespoons water. Add the chopped coriander and stir to mix well.

4 Lightly grease a 23 cm (9 inch) nonstick frying pan and place over a medium heat. Pour in a quarter of the egg mixture and swirl the pan to cover the base evenly. Cook over a gentle heat for a few minutes or until the top is just set. Remove and keep warm while you make 3 more pancakes.

5 Place each pancake on a serving plate and spoon the vegetable mixture in the centre of each one. Roll up and serve.

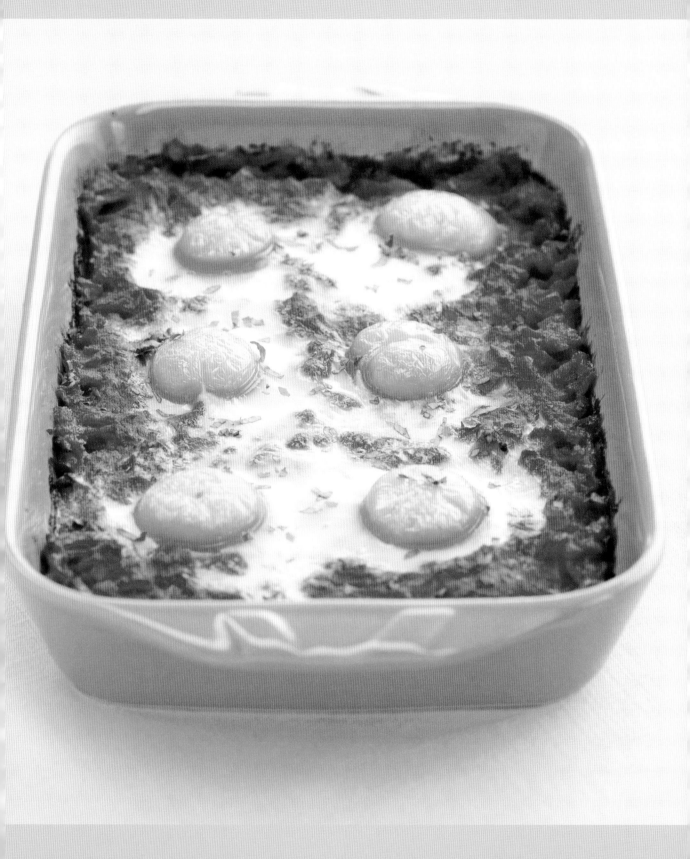

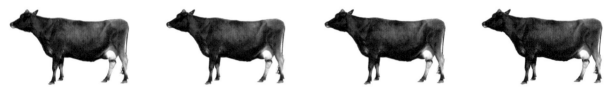

Beef

What's in it?
Lean roast beef (well done)

Nutrient	100 g (3½ oz)	28g /1¼ oz 1 thin slice
Calories	202 kcal	57 kcal
Protein	36.2 g	10.1 g
Fat	6.3 g	1.8 g
Carb	0 g	0 g
Vitamin B2	20.3 mg	0.1 mg
Vitamin B3	13.9 m	3.9 mg
Vitamin B6	0.6 mg	0.2 mg
Vitamin B12	23 mcg	0.8 mcg
Phosphorus	230 mg	64 mg
Iron	2.9 mg	0.8 mg
Zinc	6.5 mg	1.8 mg

Benefits

- Prevents anaemia
- Improves concentration and performance at school
- Helps ADHD
- Boosts immunity

Beef up mealtimes and your children will have plenty of energy to perform better – inside and outside of the classroom.

Eat to beat anaemia

Beef is packed with many nutrients including protein, phosphorus, zinc, sulphur and vitamins B2, B3, B6 and B12. But the real hero is iron, an essential part of oxygen-carrying haemoglobin in the blood. A lack of iron results in anaemia, causing tiredness, lack of energy, breathlessness, dizziness and poor concentration. Depleted iron stores and fussy eating habits make anaemia the most common dietary problem in young children. Teenage girls are also at risk of anaemia as they have higher iron requirements due to menstruation – around half of all 11–18-year-old girls have iron intakes below the minimum amount recommended for good health.

Better learning

The type of iron found in beef (haem iron) is more easily absorbed and used by the body than iron present in plant foods (non-haem iron). This makes beef a great choice for children. Numerous studies show even a mild deficiency of iron can affect a child's learning ability, while boosting intakes improves behaviour, concentration, mental sharpness and cognitive development.

Slimmer, fitter kids

According to a study in the journal *Pediatrics*, children and teenagers deficient in iron are more likely to be overweight due to overall poor eating habits. Furthermore, children with poor iron stores may feel constantly tired and therefore be less active, which can promote weight gain. Better still, lean beef can contain as little as 5 per cent fat and is not as bad for waistlines as many of us think. Plus around half the fat in beef is heart-healthy monosaturates.

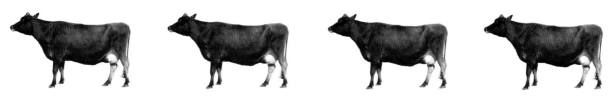

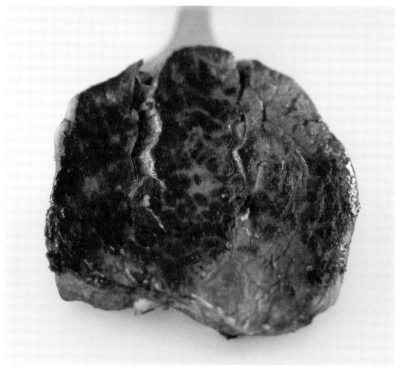

Stand to attention

New research has linked low iron intakes with Attention Deficit Hyperactivity Disorder (ADHD). A study in the medical journal *Archives of Pediatrics and Adolescent Medicine* found that 84 per cent of children with ADHD had abnormal iron stores. Furthermore, those children with the lowest iron stores had the most severe ADHD symptoms.

Prevent coughs and colds

The iron and zinc in beef help to boost immunity so children are less likely to pick up coughs and colds. According to the Common Cold Centre in the UK, low zinc levels impair the immune system and even a mild deficiency may upset the body's balance of infection-fighting white cells. Beef also contains a fatty acid called conjugated linoleic acid (CLA), which may boost immunity by making more disease-fighting white blood cells.

Looking forward

Beef contains vitamins B6 and B12. These help to lower homocysteine, high levels of which are linked to heart attacks and strokes. Plus, beef contains cancer-preventing selenium.

Won't eat...
A steak

Might eat...
Roast beef and tomato sandwich

Will eat...
Homemade burgers

Three ways
to get your kids to eat more beef

1 Mix lean minced beef with fresh tomato sauce and serve with pasta.

2 Make beef kebabs using cubes of lean beef and favourite vegetables.

3 Add small chunks of lean beef to stews, soups and casseroles.

Why not try...

Creamy beef, pea and tomato kheema (see page 96)
Nutritional facts per portion
388 kcal, 11.6 g fat (of which 4.8 g saturates), 5.4 g sugars, 0.3 g salt

Beany beef pies (see page 96)
Nutritional facts per portion
337 kcal, 13.6 g fat (of which 5.9 g saturates), 6.6 g sugars, 0.6 g salt

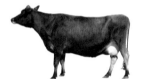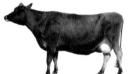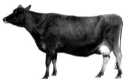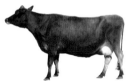

Creamy beef, pea and tomato kheema

● Preparation time **20 mins** ● Cooking time **1 hour–1 hour 10 mins** ● Serves **6**

1 tbsp **sunflower oil**
1 **red onion, finely chopped**
2 **garlic cloves, finely chopped**
1 tsp **finely grated fresh root ginger**
1 tbsp **mild curry powder**
400 g (13 oz) **lean minced beef**
400 g (13 oz) **can chopped tomatoes**
1 tsp **golden caster sugar**
200 g (7 oz) **peas (thawed if frozen)**
100 ml (3½ fl oz) **reduced-fat crème fraîche**
3–4 tbsp **fresh coriander leaves, finely chopped**
300 g **basmati rice**

1 Heat the oil in a large, nonstick saucepan over medium heat. Add the onion and stir-fry until softened, then add the garlic, ginger and curry powder and stir-fry for a further 2–3 minutes. Turn up the heat to high.

2 Add the beef, breaking it up as you do so, and fry, stirring, for 5–6 minutes until sealed and browned. Add the tomatoes and sugar, bring to the boil, reduce the heat to low, cover tightly and simmer gently for 45–50 minutes, stirring occasionally.

3 Stir in the peas and cook for a further 5–6 minutes before removing from the heat. Stir in the crème fraîche and chopped coriander and serve.

4 While the kheema is simmering, cook the rice according to the pack instructions. Serve with the kheema.

Beany beef pies

● Preparation time **30 mins** ● Cooking time **1 hour 35 mins–1 hour 50 mins** ● Serves **6**

600 g (1¼ lb) **potatoes, roughly chopped**
150 ml (¼ pint) **milk**
1 tbsp **olive oil**
1 **small onion, finely chopped**
1 **carrot, finely chopped**
1 **celery stick, finely chopped**
2 **garlic cloves, finely chopped**
500 g (1 lb) **lean minced beef**
1 tsp **ground cinnamon**
1 tsp **ground cumin**
400 g (13 oz) **can chopped tomatoes**
150 ml (¼ pint) **passata**
200 g (7 oz) **can mixed beans in water, drained**
pepper
50 g (2 oz) **Cheddar cheese, grated, to sprinkle**

1 Cook the potatoes in a large saucepan of boiling water for 12–15 minutes or until tender. Drain, return to the pan, add the milk and mash until smooth. Set aside.

2 Heat the oil in a large, heavy-based saucepan. Add the onion, carrot, celery and garlic and cook, stirring, over a medium heat for 3–4 minutes. Turn the heat to high and add the beef. Stir-fry for 4–5 minutes or until the meat is sealed and browned.

3 Add the cinnamon, cumin, tomatoes and passata and bring to the boil. Reduce the heat, cover and cook on a low heat for 45–50 minutes, stirring occasionally. Stir in the beans, season with pepper and cook for 10 minutes, until thick and hot.

4 Spoon the mince mixture into 6 individual, ovenproof pie dishes. Top each pie with the potato mixture, sprinkle over the cheese and bake in a preheated oven, 200°C (400°F), Gas Mark 6, for 20–25 minutes or until the top is lightly browned and bubbling.

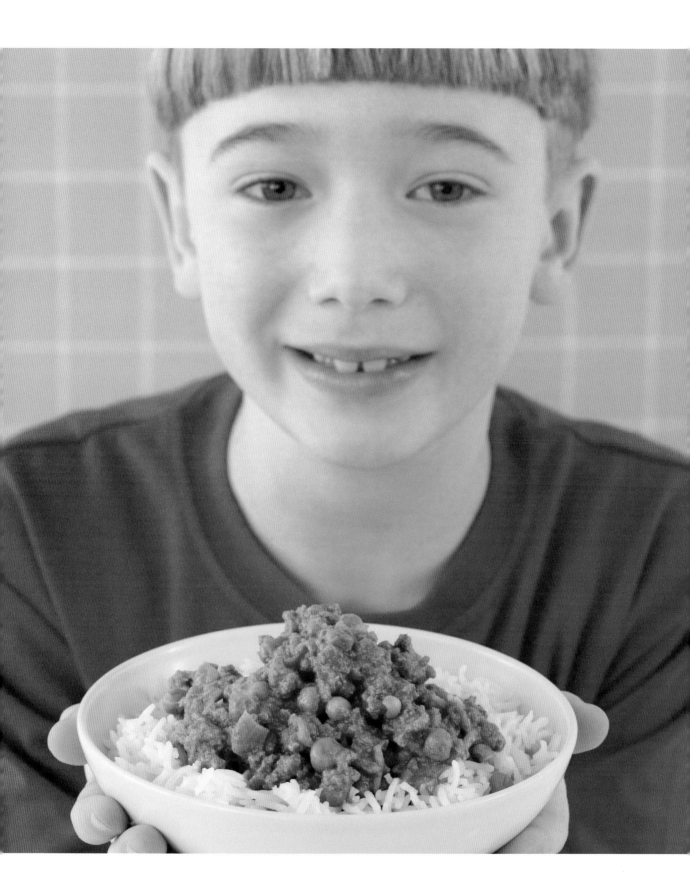

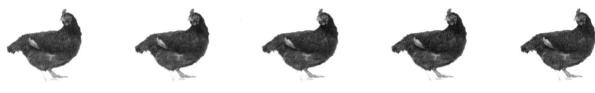

Chicken

What's in it?
Skinless roast chicken

Nutrient	100 g (3½ oz)	40 g/1¾ oz 1 slice
Calories	177 kcal	71 kcal
Protein	27.3 g	10.9 g
Fat	7.5 g	3 g
Carb	0 g	0 g
Vitamin B3	14.5 mg	5.8 mg
Vitamin B6	0.4 mg	0.11 mg
Phosphorus	220 mg	88 mg
Zinc	1.5 mg	0.6 mg
Selenium	16 mcg	6 mcg

Benefits

- **Great for cell growth and repair**
- **Boosts immunity**
- **Promotes sleep and eases stress**
- **Good for period problems**

Great for sandwiches and soups, chicken is one food children love. Fortunately, it's also packed with nutrients to keep them healthy.

Protein power

Chicken is a fabulous food for children because it is packed with B vitamins and minerals, including phosphorus, zinc, sulphur and selenium. Plus it's a great source of protein, essential for growth and the repair of cells. Because children are growing, they need more protein than adults in proportion to their size, but it's easy to meet these requirements if they eat meat, poultry, dairy products and eggs. Just one grilled chicken breast provides all the daily protein needed by an 11-year-old in order to maintain and grow healthy muscles, tendons, organs, skin and hair.

Boost immunity

Chicken is a good source of zinc, a nutrient that helps fight infection and increase resistance to coughs and colds. Unfortunately, the latest National Diet and Nutrition Survey for Young People in the UK shows that many children have low zinc intakes – for example, a third of 11–14-year-old girls have intakes below the recommended minimum and so are at risk of deficiency.

A good night's sleep

Serve chicken for dinner as it is packed with sleep-inducing tryptophan. This amino acid is used to make serotonin, a brain chemical that induces sleep.

Relieve stress

Chicken is a great food for stressed-out or anxious teenagers as it contains vitamin B5 (pantothenic acid). As well as helping to metabolise nutrients and maintain communication between the brain and nervous system, this vitamin produces stress-relieving hormones. Teenagers anxious about looming exams may be making more stress hormones and could benefit from more B5.

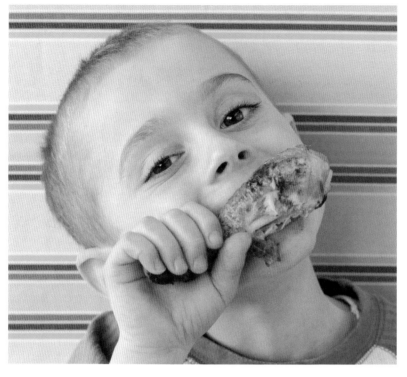

Good for period problems

Eating chicken may help teenage girls cope with the side-effects of fluctuating hormones linked to the menstrual cycle. Chicken contains vitamin B6, which may control outbreaks of acne and ease symptoms of pre-menstrual syndrome (PMS) by regulating hormone levels.

Treating autism

Boosting vitamin B6 intakes may help some autistic children. Evidence from around 20 published studies indicates that vitamin B6 was found to be beneficial in half of all subjects, although vitamin intakes were usually boosted with supplements rather than food.

Looking forward

The B vitamins in chicken keep the heart healthy. Nicotinic acid – a component of niacin (vitamin B3) – may lower cholesterol, while vitamins B6 and B12 are involved in processing homocysteine, high blood levels of which increase the risk of heart disease. Chicken also contains selenium, an antioxidant that may fight heart disease, cancer and even cataracts.

Won't eat...
Grilled chicken breast

Might eat...
Roast chicken with gravy

Will eat...
Grilled chicken in a bun with cheese and tomato

Three ways
to get your kids to eat more chicken

1 Ditch ready-made chicken nuggets and use minced chicken to make your own.

2 Use leftover roast chicken in sandwiches, salads, stir-fries and burritos, or use to top pizzas.

3 Make homemade chicken and vegetable soup, using your child's favourite vegetables.

Why not try...

Baked chicken nuggets with tomato sauce
(see page 100)
Nutritional facts per portion
251 kcal, 2.9 g fat (of which 0.4 g saturates), 3.7 g sugars, 0.9 g salt

Chicken and mixed vegetable rice (see page 100)
Nutritional facts per portion
430 kcal, 10.6 g fat (of which 2 g saturates), 4.8 g sugars, 0.6 g salt

Baked chicken nuggets with tomato sauce

● Preparation time **30 mins** ● Cooking time **30–40 mins** ● Serves **6**

Sauce:
½ **small onion**
2–3 **garlic cloves, finely chopped**
400 g (13 oz) **can chopped tomatoes**
1 tsp **golden caster sugar**
3 tbsp **finely chopped basil pepper**

Nuggets:
4 **large boneless and skinless chicken breasts**
200 g (7 oz) **dried wholemeal breadcrumbs, finely crushed**
2 tsp **dried mixed herbs**
olive oil, for brushing

1 Make the sauce. Put the onion, garlic, tomatoes and sugar in a small saucepan. Bring to the boil, reduce the heat and simmer gently for 10–15 minutes, stirring occasionally. Stir in the basil, season with pepper, set aside and keep warm.

2 Cut the chicken into bite-sized pieces. In a large bowl mix together the breadcrumbs and dried herbs.

3 Lightly brush the chicken pieces all over with olive oil. Spread the breadcrumb mixture on a flat tray and roll the chicken pieces in it to coat each piece evenly. Arrange the coated chicken pieces on a lined and greased baking sheet and bake in a preheated oven, 200°C (400°F), Gas Mark 6, for 20–25 minutes or until cooked through. Serve warm with the tomato sauce.

Chicken and mixed vegetable rice

● Preparation time **20 mins** ● Cooking time **10–14 mins** ● Serves **4**

2 tbsp **olive oil**
1 **garlic clove, finely chopped**
½ tsp **fresh root ginger, finely grated**
6 **spring onions, finely chopped**
100 g (3½ oz) **baby sweetcorn, cut into bite-sized pieces**
100 g (3½ oz) **mangetout, cut into bite-sized pieces**
1 **red pepper, deseeded and finely diced**
3 **cooked chicken breasts, skinned and roughly chopped**
200 g (7 oz) **cooked brown rice**
300 g (10 oz) **cooked white basmati or long-grain rice**
1 tsp **roasted sesame oil**
1 tbsp **reduced-salt soy sauce**

1 Heat the oil in a large, nonstick frying pan or wok. Add the garlic, ginger and spring onions and stir-fry over a medium heat for 2–3 minutes.

2 Add the sweetcorn, mangetout and red pepper and stir-fry for 2–3 minutes. Pour in about 50 ml (2 fl oz) water, stir and allow the vegetables to cook for a further 2–3 minutes.

3 Turn the heat to high and add the chicken and the rice. Stir-fry for 4–5 minutes or until the mixture is piping hot. Remove from the heat and stir in the sesame oil and soy sauce. Stir to mix and serve immediately.

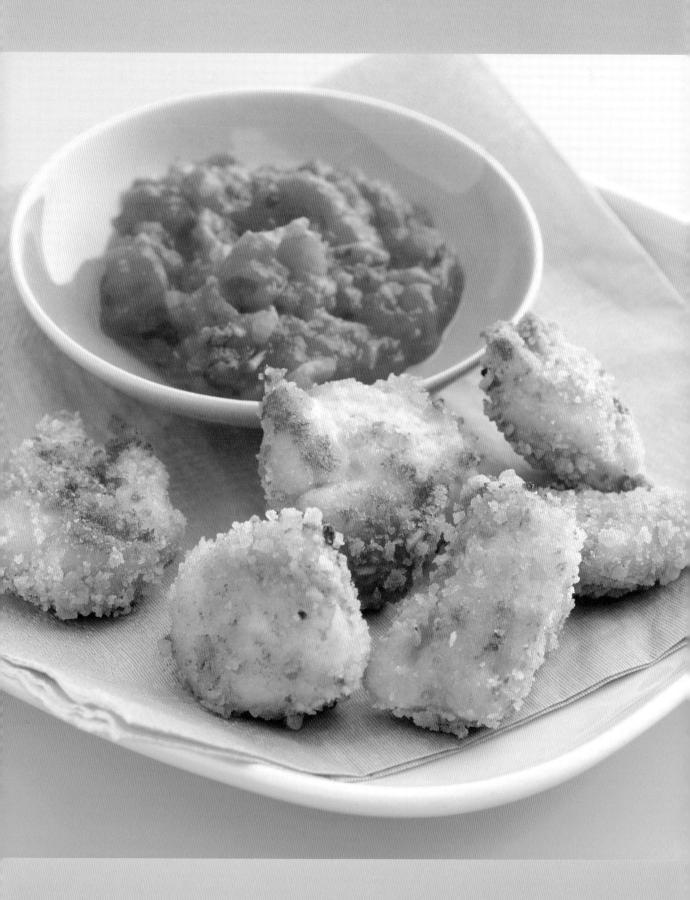

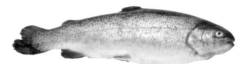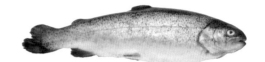

Cod

What's in it?
Baked cod with a little butter

Nutrient	100 g 3½ oz	120g/4oz cod fillet
Calories	96 kcal	115 kcal
Protein	21.4 g	25.7 g
Fat	1.2 g	1.4 g
Carb	0 g	0 g
Vitamin B3	5.7 mg	6.8 mg
Vitamin B6	0.4 mg	0.5 mg
Vitamin B12	2 mcg	2.4 mcg
Phosphorus	190 mg	228 mg
Selenium	34 mcg	41 mcg
Iodine	110 mcg	132 mcg

Benefits
- Boosts IQ
- Healthy teeth
- Great for hair, skin and nails
- Heart health

Fish fingers might be a favourite with children, but there are plenty of other reasons why you should make cod the catch of the day.

Seafood... and eat it

It's the perfect accompaniment to French fries, but there's more to cod than simply a great taste. This popular fish is packed with protein and contains good amounts of several B vitamins, phosphorus, iodine, fluoride and sulphur. Plus, it contains selenium, good intakes of which have been linked with preventing asthma (see Sunflower seeds).

Food for the body and brain

Encouraging children to eat cod is an easy way to boost intakes of iodine, a trace element that helps enhance IQ. Iodine keeps the thyroid gland healthy enabling it to make thyroxine, a hormone that regulates metabolism and promotes growth and development in children, including the brain. Iodine deficiency stunts growth and has been linked with poorer intelligence, motor skills, muscle strength, co-ordination, manual dexterity and school performance, plus learning disabilities and, in extreme cases, mental retardation. An analysis of 18 studies concluded that iodine deficiency lowers average IQ scores in children by 13.5 points. Fortunately, cod is a great food for boosting intakes – just one fillet provides all the iodine needed by teenagers for good health.

Brush up on fluoride

While toothpaste and drinking water are important sources of fluoride for children, cod can also boost levels. This nutrient strengthens the tooth enamel, making it more resistant to tooth decay. This is important because according to the most recent Children's Dental Health Survey in the UK, 38 per cent of 12-year-olds and 50 per cent of 15-year-olds have signs of tooth decay.

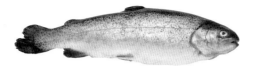
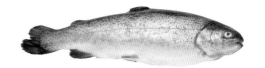

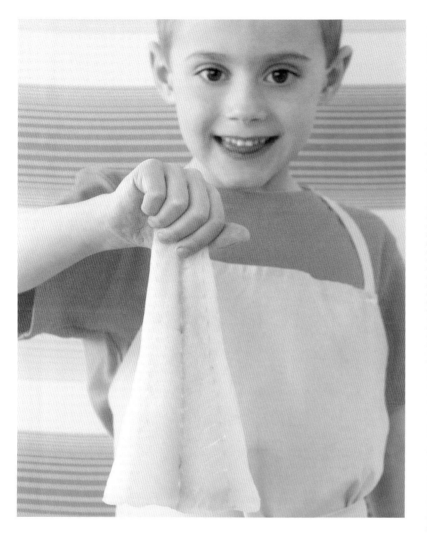

Won't eat...
Grilled cod

Might eat...
Cod with parsley sauce

Will eat...
Homemade cod fish fingers

Three ways
to get your kids to eat more cod

1 Top cod with grated cheese and place under the grill until it melts.

2 Make a Mediterranean-style fish stew using tomatoes, onions, peppers, garlic, mixed herbs and cod; serve with brown rice or couscous.

3 Make your own fish pie or fish cakes rather than relying on ready-made ones.

Why not try...
Cod and prawn pie
(see page 104)
Nutritional facts per portion
390 kcal, 15.1 g fat (of which 7 g saturates), 5.3 sugars, 1.8 g salt

Roasted cod, tomato and potato bake (see page 104)
Nutritional facts per portion
363 kcal, 7.3 g fat (of which 1 g saturates), 5.1 sugars, 0.4 g salt

Fish for compliments

Cod might not seem like the obvious ingredient for good looks, but it is packed with the 'beauty mineral', sulphur. This nutrient is present in all cells, but its greatest concentration is in hair, skin and nails. First signs of a deficiency include dry skin, brittle hair and dull, lifeless hair – not exactly what teenagers want.

A hearty meal

Cod is a great choice for a healthy heart as it is low in fat and contains vitamins B3, B6 and B12, all of which help to protect against heart disease. This is important because a Scottish study reveals that one in five children aged 11–14 years have early signs of heart disease and stroke. It also contains selenium, good intakes of which may protect against cancer.

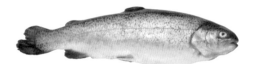
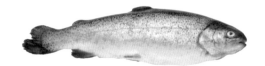

Cod and prawn pie

● Preparation time **30 mins** ● Cooking time **36–46 mins** ● Serves **4–6**

800 g (1 lb 10 oz) **potatoes, roughly chopped**

2 tbsp **unsalted butter**

75 ml (3 fl oz) **warm semi-skimmed milk**

2 tbsp **finely chopped parsley**

500 g (1 lb) **thick cod fillet, skinned**

milk, for poaching

2 tbsp **olive oil**

2 **garlic cloves, crushed**

6 **baby leeks, finely sliced**

1 **carrot, finely diced**

100 g (3½ oz) **frozen peas (thawed)**

200 ml (7 fl oz) **reduced-fat crème fraîche**

1 tsp **Dijon mustard**

1 tsp **wholegrain mustard**

200 g (7 oz) **cooked peeled prawns**

2 tbsp **chives, finely chopped**

pepper

1 Cook the potatoes in a large saucepan of boiling water for 15–20 minutes until tender. Drain, return to the pan and mash until smooth. Stir in the butter, milk and parsley and mix well to combine. Set aside and keep warm.

2 Meanwhile, place the fish in a large saucepan and cover with milk. Poach the fish for 8–10 minutes or until just cooked through, remove from the pan with a slotted spoon and break up into large flakes. Set aside.

3 Heat the oil in a large, nonstick frying pan. Add the garlic, leeks, carrot and peas, stir to mix and cook over a gentle heat for 10–12 minutes or until the carrots and leeks are tender. Add the crème fraîche, mustards and chives. Season with pepper. Stir and cook for 2–3 minutes. Add the fish and prawns and toss to coat well. Spoon this mixture into an ovenproof pie dish and spread over the topping mixture. Place under a hot grill for 3–4 minutes or until the top is golden. Serve immediately.

Roasted cod, tomato and potato bake

● Preparation time **30 mins** ● Cooking time **1½ hours** ● Serves **4**

800 g (1 lb 10 oz) **potatoes, thinly sliced**

250 ml (8 fl oz) **homemade, fat-free vegetable stock**

400 g (13 oz) **can chopped tomatoes**

2–3 **garlic cloves, crushed**

1 tsp **dried oregano**

2 tbsp **olive oil**

1 tsp **golden caster sugar**

4 **thick cod fillets, skinned and cut into large chunks**

pepper

chopped flat leaf parsley

1 Layer the potatoes in the base of a lightly greased, medium-sized, ovenproof dish. Add the stock, cover with foil and bake in a preheated oven, 190°C (375°F), Gas Mark 5, for 30 minutes or until the stock is almost absorbed.

2 Mix together the tomatoes with the garlic, oregano, olive oil and sugar, season with pepper and spoon this mixture over the potatoes. Return to the oven and bake for a further 30 minutes.

3 Remove the dish from the oven and arrange the fish over the top in a single layer. Season and return to the oven for 20–25 minutes or until the fish is cooked through. Remove from the oven, scatter over the parsley and serve.

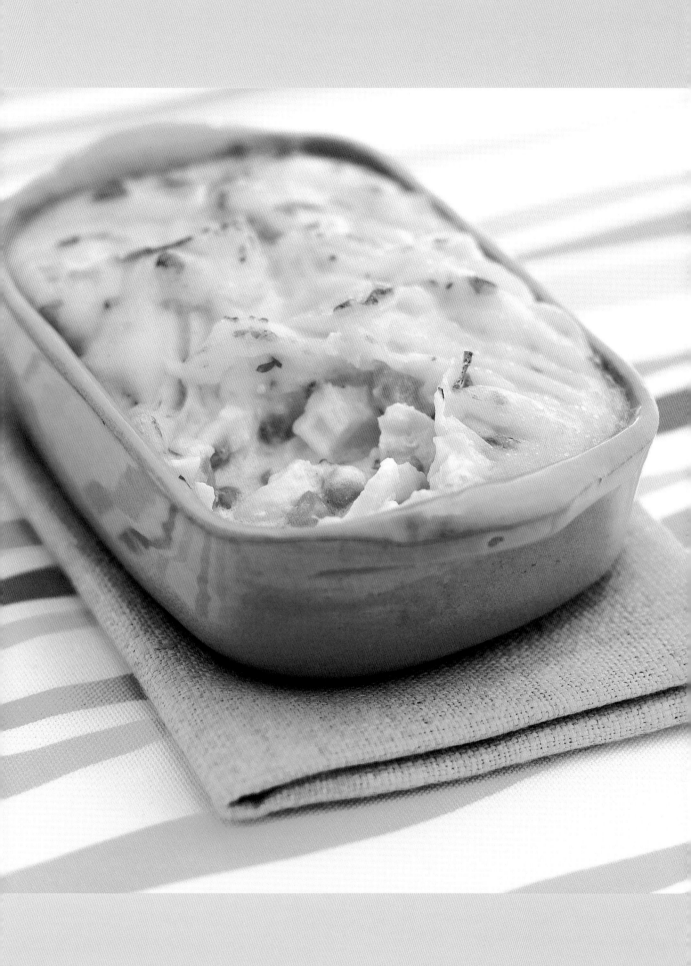

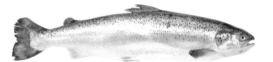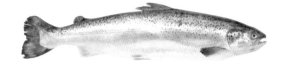

Salmon

It can boost brain power, improve behaviour and ease allergies. No wonder salmon is such a great choice for kids.

What's in it?
Canned Pacific salmon in water

Nutrient	100 g (3½ oz)	50 g/2 oz serving
Calories	153 kcal	77 kcal
Protein	23.5 g	11.8 g
Fat	6.6 g	3.3 g
Carb	0 g	0 g
Vitamin B3	10.3 mg	5.2 mg
Vitamin B6	0.2 mg	0.1 mg
Vitamin B12	4 mcg	2 mcg
Vitamin D	9.2 mcg	4.6 mcg
Vitamin E	1.5 mg	0.8 mg
Phosphorus	170 mg	85 mg
Iron	0.6 mg	0.3 mg
Selenium	25 mcg	13 mcg
Iodine	59 mcg	30 mcg

Benefits
- Boosts brain power
- Improves behavioural problems
- Eases allergies
- Prevents blood clots, stroke and heart attacks

Superfood salmon

Salmon is packed with protein and contains iron, phosphorus, selenium, iodine and sulphur together with a range of B vitamins and vitamins D and E. But its omega-3 fats – a type of polyunsaturated fat – are what give salmon its superfood status. Research shows that while most children are meeting guidelines for intakes of polyunsaturates, they are having insufficient omega-3s and too many omega-6s (another polyunsaturated fat found mainly in vegetable oils and margarines). This may cause health problems later in life, but can easily be prevented by eating more omega-3-rich salmon. Children should eat at least one serving of oily fish a week, but girls shouldn't have more than two servings weekly as oily fish can be contaminated with pollutants that are stored in the body and can affect a developing baby (see Introduction).

Brain food

Salmon is the ultimate brain food. Almost two-thirds of the brain consists of fat, with half of this being omega-3s. At birth, more than three-quarters of the cells that will ever be present in the brain have already formed, so it is vital for mothers to eat plenty of omega-3 rich foods when pregnant. The remaining cells are formed in the first few years of life and then get bigger as children grow and learn new things. So if you want brainy kids, get them eating oily fish, especially when they're young.

Food for behaviour therapy

Eating more oily fish may improve Attention Deficit Hyperactivity Disorder (ADHD), dyslexia and dyspraxia (clumsiness). Research shows low omega-3 intakes are linked to hyperactivity, learning difficulties, behavioural problems and temper tantrums in

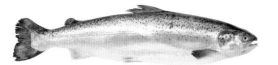
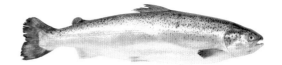

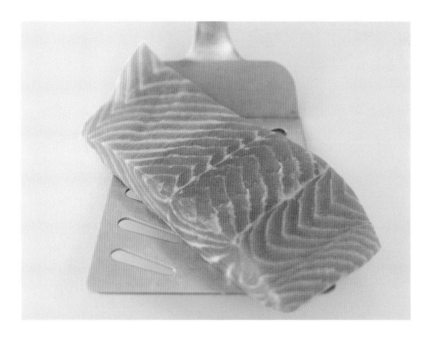

children, while boosting intakes has been shown to reduce behavioural problems and improve reading ability and dyspraxia. Omega-3 supplements may even improve language and learning skills in children with autism, although more research is needed to confirm this.

Alleviating asthma

Salmon is a great food for asthmatic children. Australian research has found that regularly consuming oily fish reduces the chances of developing asthma in childhood. In a study of 8–11-year-olds, those who ate oily fish were four times less likely to develop asthma than those who never ate it. The reason: omega-3s make hormone-like substances called prostaglandins that help reduce inflammation in the lungs.

Easing eczema

Research shows that eczema sufferers often have low levels of omega-3s, so encouraging children with eczema to eat salmon may help reduce the inflammation and severity of this skin condition.

Looking forward

In adults, omega-3s may prevent heart attacks, blood clots, strokes, depression and Alzheimer's disease, and improve the symptoms of rheumatoid arthritis and lupus.

Won't eat...
A salmon steak

Might eat...
Salmon fish pie

Will eat...
Salmon fishcakes

Three ways
to get your kids to eat more salmon

1 Replace tuna, chicken or ham with canned Pacific salmon in salads, sandwiches and baked potatoes.

2 Mix canned Pacific salmon with cooked pasta, sweetcorn and soft cheese and heat through for a nutritious meal.

3 Make salmon kebabs and serve with pitta and a yogurt dip.

Why not try...

Salmon fishcakes with minted mushy peas
(see page 108)
Nutritional facts per fishcakes
102 kcal, 5 g fat (of which 0.9 g saturates), 0.8 g sugars, 0.1 g salt

Teriyaki salmon
(see page 108)
Nutritional facts per portion
331 kcal, 18.7 g fat (of which 3.2 g saturates), 0.1 g sugars, 0.9 g salt

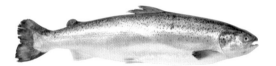
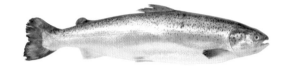

Salmon fishcakes with minted mushy peas

● Preparation time **30 mins, plus chilling** ● Cooking time **32–43 mins** ● Makes **16**

600 g (1¼ lb) **potatoes, roughly chopped**
2 **garlic cloves, crushed**
6 **spring onions, finely sliced**
2 tbsp **finely chopped flat leaf parsley**
¼ tsp **finely grated fresh root ginger**
400 g (13 oz) **salmon fillet, skinned and roughly chopped**
2 tsp **Dijon mustard**
2 tbsp **mayonnaise**
olive oil, for brushing
Mushy peas:
200 g (7 oz) **peas (thawed if frozen)**
2 tbsp **reduced-fat crème fraîche**
1 tbsp **finely chopped mint leaves**
pepper

1 Cook the potatoes in a large saucepan of boiling water for 15–20 minutes until tender. Drain, return to the pan and mash until fairly smooth. Transfer to a large mixing bowl and set aside.

2 Place the garlic, spring onions, parsley, ginger and salmon in a food processor or blender and process until well mixed. Add the fish to the potatoes, mustard and mayonnaise. Use your fingers to combine the mixture evenly. Divide the mixture into 16 portions and form each one into a flat cake. Grease and line a baking sheet. Space the fishcakes on the baking sheet, cover and chill for 30–40 minutes.

3 Brush the fishcakes with olive oil and bake in a preheated oven, 190°C (375°F), Gas Mark 5, for 15–20 minutes or until the cakes are lightly browned and cooked through. Remove from the oven and keep warm.

4 Meanwhile, make the mushy peas. Boil the peas in boiling water for 2–3 minutes. Drain and place in a food processor or blender with the crème fraîche and mint. Season with pepper and process until fairly smooth. Transfer to a small saucepan and keep warm until ready to serve with the fishcakes.

Teriyaki salmon

● Preparation time **20 mins, plus marinating** ● Cooking time **6–8 mins** ● Serves **4**

600 g (1¼ lb) **thick salmon fillet, skinned**
2 tbsp **clear honey**
1 tbsp **reduced-salt dark soy sauce**
2 tbsp **tomato ketchup**
1 tsp **sesame oil**
½ tsp **finely grated fresh root ginger**
2 tsp **roasted sesame seeds**

1 Cut the salmon into bite-sized pieces and place them on a shallow dish in a single layer.

2 In a small bowl mix together the honey, soy sauce, ketchup, sesame oil and ginger until well combined. Pour this mixture over the salmon and toss to coat evenly. Cover and marinate in the refrigerator for 20–30 minutes.

3 Place the salmon pieces in a single layer on a lightly oiled grill pan. Cook under a medium-hot grill for 6–8 minutes or until cooked to your liking. Carefully remove from the grill, sprinkle over the sesame seeds and serve immediately.

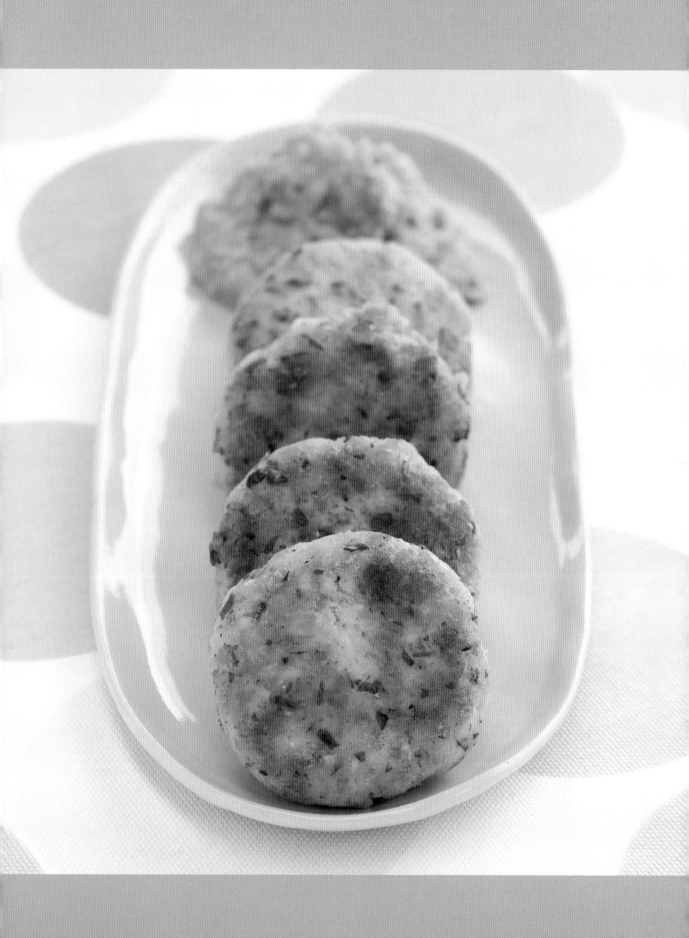

Kidney beans

Kidney beans are a great addition to kid's diets – providing short- and long-term health benefits, thanks to their unique combination of nutrients.

What's in them?
Canned kidney beans (drained)

Nutrient	100 g (3½ oz)	35g / 1½ oz 1 tbsp
Calories	100 kcal	35 kcal
Protein	6.9 g	2.4 g
Fat	0.6 g	0.2 g
Carb	17.8 g	6.2 g
Fibre	6.2 g	2.2 g
Vitamin B1	0.2 mg	0.1 mg
Phosphorus	130 mg	46 mg
Potassium	280 mg	98 mg
Iron	2 mg	0.7 mg

Benefits
- May benefit asthmatics
- Good protein source for vegetarians
- Boost memory
- Prevent obesity, diabetes and heart disease

Beneficial beans

Pulses are a great food for children as they are packed with energy-boosting carbohydrates, filling fibre and protein for growth. Plus they contain health-promoting vitamins and minerals, including vitamin B1, folate, phosphorus, potassium and iron. Canned pulses contain similar nutrients to dried ones and are far more convenient, although opt for those canned without added salt or sugar.

Breathe easy

Kidney beans may be particularly beneficial for children who suffer with asthma as they contain good amounts of molybdenum. This mineral is an essential ingredient for the enzyme sulphite oxidase, which destroys sulphites. Sulphites are used as a preservative in many foods typically eaten by children, such as soft drinks, sausages and burgers – look out for E220 to E228 on ingredients lists. The US Food and Drug Administration estimates that around 5 per cent of asthmatics are sensitive to sulphites, although an allergy expert in Australia estimates that this figure could be as high as 20 per cent. Adding kidney beans to your child's diet will boost low molybdenum levels, which in turn will make more of the enzyme that destroys sulphites.

Great for vegetarians

According to the latest UK National Diet and Nutrition Survey of Young People, one in ten girls aged 15–18 is vegetarian. Kidney beans can make an important contribution to vegetarian diets as they contain reasonable amounts of iron, a nutrient that is often lacking due to the exclusion of meat (see Beef). And when eaten with other plant foods, they provide all the

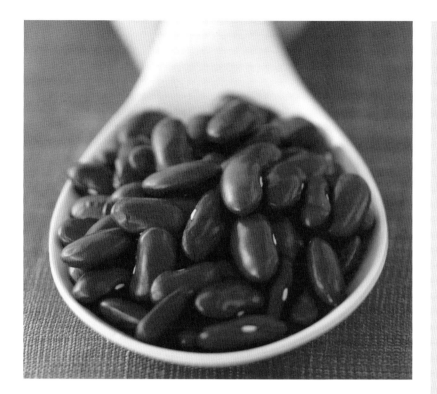

essential amino acids (protein building-blocks) needed for good health. Like peas, beans lack an essential amino acid called methionine but contain good amounts of the essential amino acid lysine. In contrast, cereals such as rice contain methionine but lack lysine. This means that it is a good idea for vegetarian children to eat plant foods together, for example, combining vegetable chilli with rice.

Be a brain box

Encouraging children to eat kidney beans may help them perform better in tests and exams. Research shows that a deficiency in vitamin B1 (thiamin) – found in good amounts in kidney beans – can result in a poor memory. As well as converting carbohydrates into energy that is used by brain cells, this vitamin makes the neurotransmitter acetylcholine, which is essential for memory.

Looking forward

Like all pulses, kidney beans contain soluble fibre. This helps to keep blood-sugar levels steady, in the long term preventing obesity and diabetes, and lowering cholesterol.

Won't eat...
Kidney beans as an accompaniment

Might eat...
Kidney beans mixed with baked beans

Will eat...
Mild chilli in pitta bread with grated cheese

Three ways
to get your kids to eat more kidney beans

1 Add kidney beans to stews, casseroles and soups; try puréeing soups for a creamy texture.

2 Make a dip by mashing kidney beans with a little olive oil, garlic and chilli powder.

3 For a tasty baked potato topping, mix kidney beans with tuna, diced peppers and reduced-fat mayonnaise.

Why not try...

Mini spiced bean burgers with kachumber (see page 112)
Nutritional facts per portion
151 kcal, 3.9 g fat (of which 0.6 g saturates), 3.1 g sugars, 0.4 g salt

Sausage and bean stew
(see page 112)
Nutritional facts per portion
239 kcal, 9.6 g fat (of which 2.5 g saturates), 10.4 g sugars, 1.4 g salt

Mini spiced bean burgers

● Preparation time **30 mins, plus chilling** ● Cooking time **about 30 mins** ● Makes **12**

1 small cucumber, finely diced
2 ripe tomatoes, finely diced
¼ red onion, finely diced
large handful of mint leaves,
    finely chopped
385 g (12½ oz) can red kidney
    beans, rinsed and drained
1 garlic clove, crushed
1 tsp finely grated fresh
    root ginger
1 tsp roasted cumin seeds
1 tsp mild curry powder
2 tbsp finely chopped
    fresh coriander leaves
1 small egg, lightly beaten
200 g (7 oz) mashed potato
flour, for dusting
3 tbsp sunflower oil
wholemeal pitta bread

1 Combine the cucumber, tomatoes, red onion and mint in a bowl, mix well, cover and chill until ready to use.

2 Put the beans, garlic, ginger, cumin seeds, curry powder, coriander leaves and egg in a food processor or blender. Process until fairly smooth and transfer to a bowl. Add the mashed potato and use your fingers to mix until thoroughly combined. Divide the mixture into 12 portions and form each one into a flat burger. Grease and line a baking sheet. Space the burgers on the baking sheet, cover and chill for 3–4 hours or overnight if time permits.

3 Lightly dust the burgers with flour. Heat the oil in a large, nonstick frying pan and cook the burgers, in batches, for 5–6 minutes, turning once, until lightly golden.

4 Serve each burger with the cucumber dip and half a toasted wholemeal pitta bread.

Sausage and bean stew

● Preparation time **20 minutes** ● Cooking time **50–60 mins** ● Serves **6**

6 reduced-fat pork sausages
2 tbsp olive oil
1 onion, finely chopped
2 garlic cloves, crushed
1 bay leaf
1 carrot, finely chopped
1 celery stick, finely chopped
2 tsp dried thyme
400 g (13 oz) can chopped
    tomatoes
200 ml (7 fl oz) passata
2 tsp golden caster sugar
2 x 385 g (12½ oz) cans red
    kidney beans, drained
pepper

1 Put the sausages under a medium grill and cook until lightly browned. Remove and set aside.

2 Meanwhile, heat the oil over a medium heat in a nonstick saucepan. Add the onion, garlic, bay leaf, carrot and celery and stir-fry for 4–5 minutes.

3 Sprinkle in the thyme, add the tomatoes, passata and sugar and bring the mixture to the boil. Cover, reduce the heat and allow to cook on a low heat for 30–40 minutes, stirring occasionally.

4 Cut the sausages into bite-sized pieces and add to the hotpot with the beans. Season with pepper and cook for 3–4 minutes or until piping hot.

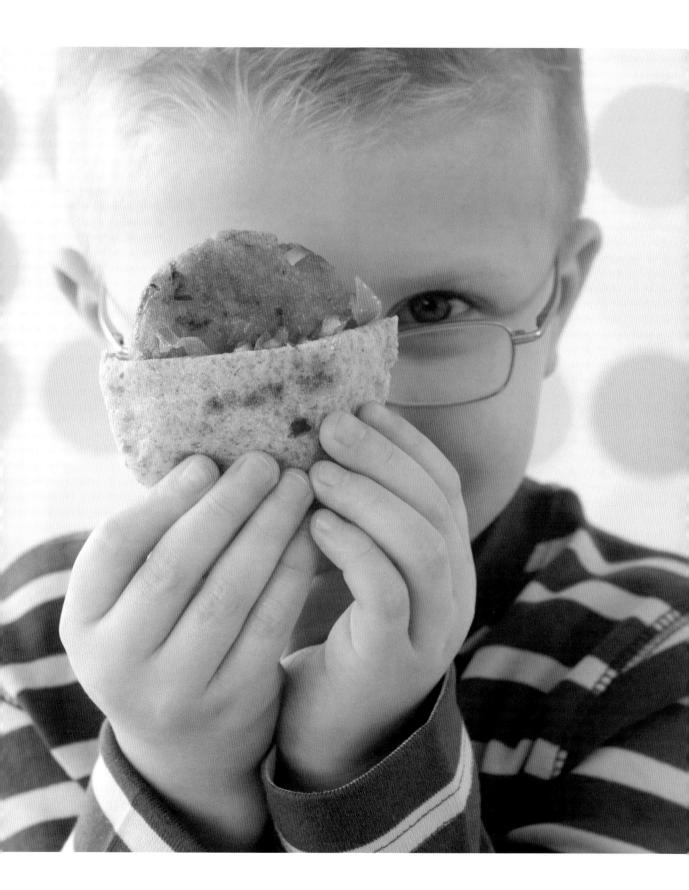

Sunflower seeds

What's in them?
Sunflower seeds

Nutrient	100 g (3½ oz)	20g /¾ oz 1 tbsp
Calories	581 kcal	93 kcal
Protein	19.8 g	3.2 g
Fat	47.5 g	7.6 g
Carb	18.6 g	3 g
Fibre	6 g	1 g
Vitamin B1	1.6 mg	0.3 mg
Vitamin B3	9.1 mg	1.5 mg
Vitamin E	37.8 mg	6 mg
Calcium	110 mg	18 mg
Phosphorus	640 mg	102 mg
Magnesium	390 mg	62 mg
Potassium	710 mg	114 mg
Iron	6.4 mg	1 mg
Zinc	5.1 mg	0.8 mg
Selenium	49 mcg	8 mcg

Benefits
- Ease asthma
- Strong bones
- Relieve stress
- Great for skin

Snacking on sunflower seeds has many benefits for kids – from easing asthma and keeping skin glowing to reducing stress and building stronger bones.

Easing asthma

Sunflower seeds are a great choice for asthmatic children as they are rich in selenium, magnesium and vitamin E, all of which have been linked with treating this disease. Magnesium relaxes the muscles in the lungs, making breathing easier. Good intakes of vitamin E have been linked with a lower risk of developing asthma and improved lung function. And research shows that children with low selenium levels are more likely to develop asthma than those with higher levels. More research is needed to confirm these benefits, but it won't hurt to encourage your children to eat sunflower seeds. Remember not to give them to children under five because of the risk of choking (see Introduction).

Pre-exam stress relief

Snacking on sunflower seeds while revising and before exams may help calm children's nerves and allow them to sleep better, thanks to muscle-relaxing magnesium. Studies show a deficiency in magnesium is linked to insomnia, while diets high in magnesium are associated with good-quality sleep. Sadly, figures from the UK's latest National Diet and Nutrition Survey of Young People show that more than half of all girls aged 11–18, more than a quarter of boys aged 11–14 and one in five boys aged 15–18 have magnesium intakes below the minimum amount recommended for good health. Sunflower seeds are also rich in vitamins B1 and B3, which are important for a healthy nervous system and have been linked with mental well-being.

Good for bones

A handful of sunflower seeds contains reasonable amounts of bone-strengthening phosphorus, although the latter is less well absorbed by the body than the calcium in dairy products (see Milk).

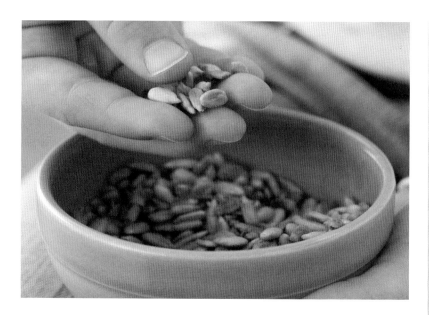

Looking good

Snacking on copper-rich sunflower seeds may keep teenager's skin and hair looking healthy. This trace mineral is important for a healthy heart, fertility and a strong immune and nervous system. But copper is also needed to make melanin – a dark, natural colour found in the hair, skin and eyes – and so helps to keep pigmentation consistent.

Great for vegetarians

Sunflower seeds can make an important contribution to vegetarian diets as they contain many nutrients typically found in meat and fish, such as protein, iron and zinc.

Super skin

Sunflower seeds are packed with skin-healthy vitamin E (see Avocado). Sunflower seeds also contain essential omega-6 fatty acids. Together with omega-3 fats, good intakes may improve inflammatory skin conditions such as eczema and psoriasis. However, it is equally important that children have good intakes of omega-3 fats (see Salmon).

Looking forward

Sunflower seeds contain antioxidants selenium and vitamin E, for protection against cancer and heart disease. They also contain naturally occurring plant compounds that reduce cholesterol.

Won't eat...
A handful of sunflower seeds

Might eat...
Homemade cereal bar containing sunflower seeds

Will eat...
Fruit crumble and custard (with sunflower seeds added to the crumble mix)

Three ways
to get your kids to eat more sunflower seeds

1 Add sunflower seeds to breakfast cereals.

2 Top salads and stir-fries with sunflower seeds to add crunch and taste.

3 Make your own seedy bread by adding a selection of seeds.

Why not try...

Sunflower and date muesli squares (see page 116)
Nutritional facts per square
204 kcal, 10.7 g fat (of which 4.4 g saturates), 14.2 g sugars, 0.2 g salt

Banana and sunflower seed bread (see page 116)
Nutritional facts per slice
195 kcal, 5.4 g fat (of which 0.7 g saturates), 12.8 g sugars, 0 g salt

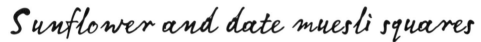

Sunflower and date muesli squares

● Preparation time **20 mins** ● Cooking time **40–50 mins** ● Makes **16**

175 g (6 oz) **dried dates, roughly chopped**
200 ml (7 fl oz) **water**
125 g (4 oz) **porridge oats**
3 tbsp **sunflower seeds**
125 g (4 oz) **wholemeal flour**
100 g (3½ oz) **light muscovado sugar**
1 tsp **baking powder**
50 g (2 oz) **chopped hazelnuts**
125 g (4 oz) **unsalted butter, softened**

1 Place the dates and water in a saucepan and bring to the boil. Reduce the heat and simmer gently for 20–25 minutes or until the dates are tender and most of the liquid is absorbed. Blend the dates in a food processor or blender until smooth. Set aside.

2 Grease and base-line a 28 x 18 cm (11 x 7 inch) baking tin. Put the porridge oats, sunflower seeds, flour, sugar, baking powder and hazelnuts in a mixing bowl and mix well. Add the butter and combine into the mixture with your fingertips until well mixed.

3 Place three-quarters of the mixture into the tin and press down to make a smooth, even layer. Spread the date mixture over in an even layer. Sprinkle over the remaining oat mixture and press down lightly. Cook in a preheated oven, 180°C (350°F), Gas Mark 4, for 20–25 minutes.

4 Allow to cool in the tin, then cut into squares and serve.

Banana and sunflower seed bread

● Preparation time **40 mins, plus proving** ● Cooking time **40–45 mins** ● Makes **12 slices**

150 g (5 oz) **wholemeal flour**
150 g (5 oz) **strong white flour**
2 sachets **easy-blend yeast**
60 g (2¼ oz) **golden caster sugar**
2 tsp **ground cinnamon**
1 tsp **allspice**
1 tsp **ground ginger**
4 **ripe bananas, mashed**
100 g (3½ oz) **sunflower seeds**
1 **large egg and 1 large egg white, beaten together**
sunflower oil, to grease

1 Sift the flours into a large mixing bowl. Sprinkle over the yeast, sugar, cinnamon, allspice, ginger and stir to mix. Add the bananas, sunflower seeds and egg. Pour 75 ml (3 fl oz) luke-warm water into the centre of the bowl and stir to form a dough.

3 Turn out the dough on a lightly floured surface and knead for 6–8 minutes until smooth. Form the dough into a ball and place in a lightly greased bowl. Cover with clingfilm and leave to rise in a warm place for 2–3 hours or until doubled in size.

4 Grease and base-line a medium-sized loaf tin. Turn out the dough on a lightly floured surface and knead for 1–2 minutes. Roll into shape and place in the tin. Cover and leave to rise for 45 minutes.

5 Bake the loaf in a preheated oven, 200°C (400°F), Gas Mark 6, for 40–45 minutes or until browned on the top. Allow to stand for 15–20 minutes on a wire rack before turning out.

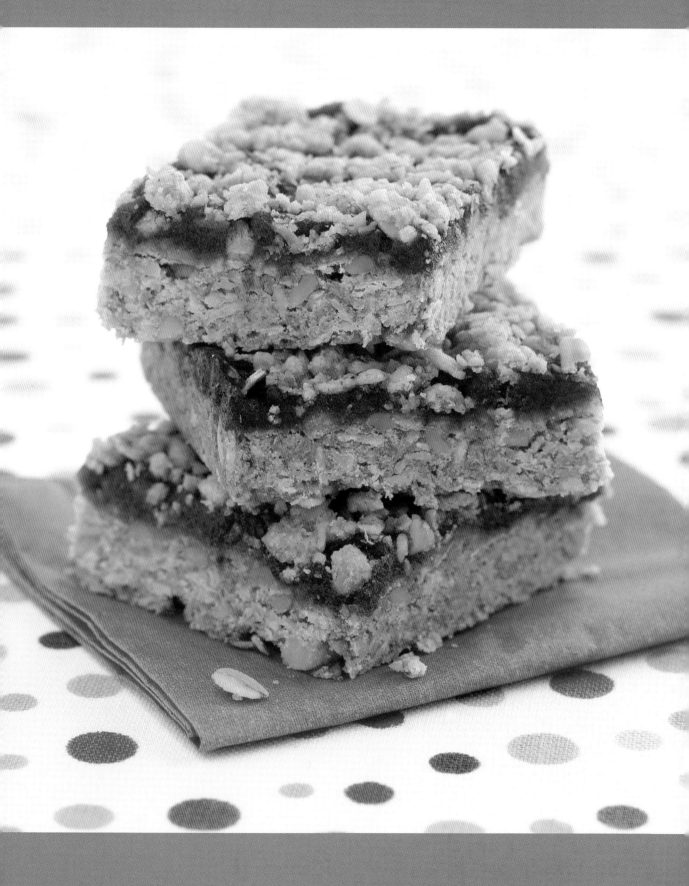

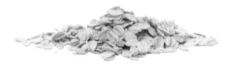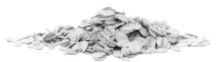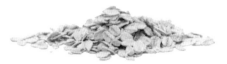

Oats

What's in them?
Cooked oats

Nutrient	100 g (3½ oz)	15g /½ oz 1 tbsp
Calories	375 kcal	56 kcal
Protein	11.2 g	1.7 g
Fat	9.2 g	1.4 g
Carb	66 g	10 g
Fibre	7.1 g	1.1 g
Vitamin B1	0.9 mg	0.1 mg
Vitamin B3	3.4 mg	0.5 mg
Vitamin E	1.5 mg	0.2 mg
Phosphorus	380 mg	57 mg
Magnesium	110 mg	17 mg
Iron	3.8 mg	0.6 mg
Zinc	3.3 mg	0.5 mg

Benefits
- Keep blood-sugar levels steady
- Maintain weight
- Boost mood and learning ability
- Lower cholesterol

For a healthy start to the day, make your kids porridge for breakfast or give them homemade oaty flapjacks to snack on after school.

Beat snack attacks

Oats contain loads of different vitamins and minerals that children need to stay healthy. Best of all, adding oats to your child's diet is a great way to satisfy their tastebuds, hunger and desire for sugary foods. Oats contain soluble fibre and have a low glycaemic index (GI). This means oats help to keep blood-sugar levels steady, preventing massive highs and lows that cause cravings for sugary and processed carbs – and constant pestering for biscuits, chocolate and sweets.

Control weight

Keeping blood-sugar levels steady also helps children control their weight by beating hunger. Research shows that oats promote satiety, too, helping children to stay fuller for longer after eating. This is an important issue since the findings from the 2004 Health Survey for England found that 33 per cent of boys and 35 per cent of girls aged 2–15 are overweight or obese.

Boost concentration

Getting children to eat porridge for breakfast may help them with their studies. Children who eat breakfast are less likely to struggle with problem-solving and perform better in mathematical and creative tasks. The type of breakfast your kids eat is also important. In a recent study, researchers from Tufts University found that children performed better after eating oatmeal compared with a sugary cereal. This is probably because carbohydrate-rich foods such as oats release glucose – the preferred fuel for the brain – steadily. Satisfied children are also more likely to be concentrating on lessons rather than grumbling tummies.

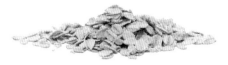
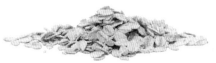
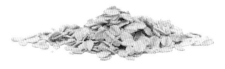

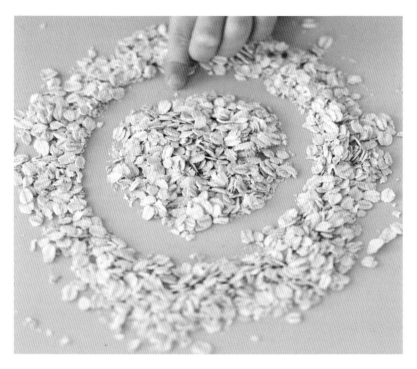

Great for kids with diabetes

Thanks to oats' ability to help control blood-sugar levels, oats are a great choice for children and teenagers with diabetes, a condition that affects around 20,000 under 15-year-olds in the UK.

Stay happy

Kids who eat oats may even be happier. Foods high in starchy carbohydrates, such as oats, boost brain levels of feel-good chemical serotonin, helping moody teenagers to beat the blues.

Good for gluten intolerance

Though oats contain gluten, a recent study of children with coeliac disease found that after a year of following a standard gluten-free diet that still included oats, the lining of the small bowel, which is damaged by wheat gluten, had healed. Always seek your doctor's advice first, if your child is intolerant to gluten.

Looking forward

The soluble fibre in oats helps to lower blood cholesterol levels, which in turn lowers the risk of heart disease and stroke. Oats also contain the plant compounds avenanthramides, which act as antioxidants.

Won't eat...
A bowl of homemade porridge

Might eat...
A bowl of instant oat cereal

Will eat...
A homemade oaty flapjack

Three ways
to get your kids to eat more oats

1 Make your own fruit and oat cookies or muffins – kids will love making them, too.

2 Encourage teenagers to eat homemade muesli instead of sugary cereals; combine oats with bran flakes, dried fruit and nuts.

3 Add oats to the crumble topping for homemade fruit crumble and serve with custard.

Why not try...

Banana and maple cinnamon porridge
(see page 120)
Nutritional facts per portion
352 kcal, 7.3 g fat (of which 1.5 g saturates), 21.8 g sugars, 0.2 g salt

Nutty raisin and oat flapjacks (see page 120)
Nutritional facts per slice
222 kcal, 12.8 g fat, (of which 2.3 g saturates), 11.3 g sugars, 0.3 g salt

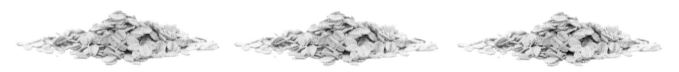

Banana and maple cinnamon porridge

● Preparation time **10 mins** ● Cooking time **5–7 mins** ● Serves **4**

225 g (7½ oz) **rolled oats**
550 ml (19 fl oz) **semi-skimmed milk**
2 **ripe bananas, sliced**
1 tsp **ground cinnamon**
4 tsp **maple syrup**

1 Place the oats and milk or water in a saucepan and bring to the boil, stirring often, to encourage the porridge to thicken. Stir and cook for 5–7 minutes or until thick and then remove from the heat.

2 Ladle the porridge into 4 warm bowls and top with the sliced banana. Sprinkle over the cinnamon and drizzle over the maple syrup before serving.

Nutty raisin and oat flapjacks

● Preparation time **15 mins** ● Cooking time **15–20 mins** ● Makes **9**

3 tbsp **self-raising flour**
3 tbsp **golden caster sugar**
100 g (3½ oz) **porridge oats**
1 tbsp **raisins**
2 tbsp **pumpkin seeds**
1 tbsp **chopped mixed nuts**
100 g (3½ oz) **unsalted butter**
1 tbsp **golden syrup**

1 Lightly grease a nonstick, 18 cm (7 inch) square, baking tin. Place the flour, sugar, oats, raisins, pumpkin seeds and chopped nuts in a large mixing bowl and stir to mix well.

2 Place the butter and golden syrup in a small saucepan and heat gently, stirring, until the butter has melted. Pour this into the oat mixture and stir to mix well.

3 Spoon the mixture into the prepared tin, pressing it down firmly to make an even layer. Cook in a preheated oven, 200°C (400°F), Gas Mark 6, for 15–20 minutes. Remove from the oven and, while still hot, carefully cut the mixture into 9 squares. Leave to cool before removing the flapjacks from the tin.

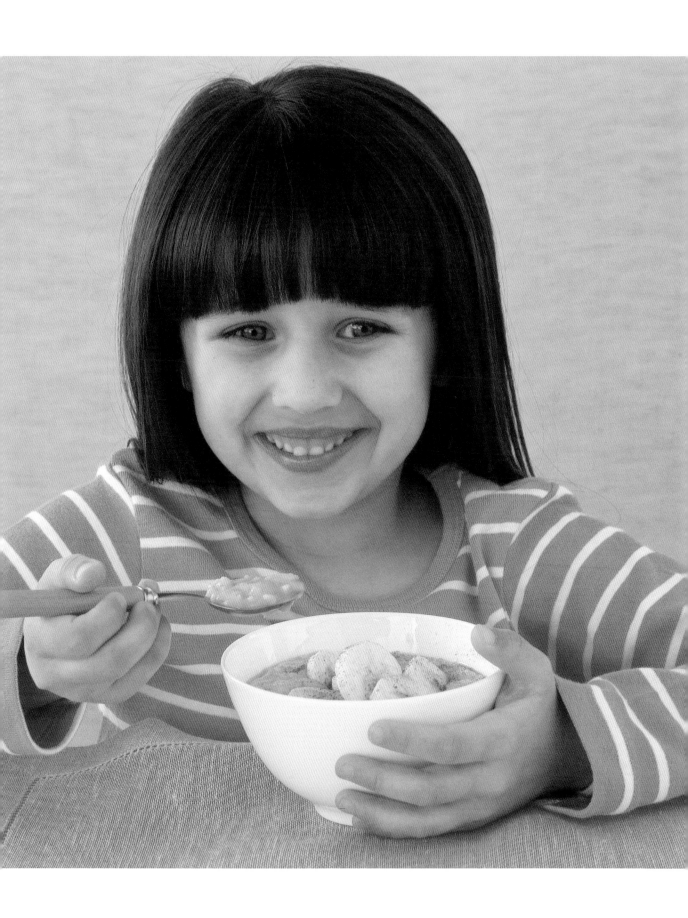

Brown rice

What's in it?
Cooked brown rice

Nutrient	100 g (3½ oz)	30g /1½ oz 1 tbsp
Calories	141 kcal	42 kcal
Protein	2.6 g	0.8 g
Fat	1.1 g	0.3 g
Carb	32.1 g	9.6 g
Fibre	0.8 g	0.2 g
Vitamin B1	0.14 mg	0.04 mg
Phosphorus	120 mg	36 mg
Magnesium	43 mg	13 mg
Manganese	0.9 mg	0.3 mg

Benefits
- Helps with sleep
- Prevents constipation
- Eases asthma
- Prevents cancer, heart disease, diabetes and obesity

Switching white rice for brown could help children sleep better and beat two common childhood complaints – constipation and asthma.

Rice that's nice

It's the perfect accompaniment to curries, chillies and stir-fries but the type of rice you serve can make a big difference to the nutritional value of a meal. The processing that converts brown into white rice removes vitamins, minerals and fibre, leaving behind a grain with few nutrients. Swapping white for brown at mealtimes will significantly boost your child's intake of fibre, vitamin B1 and minerals such as magnesium, phosphorus, copper and manganese.

Eat well, sleep well

Giving your kids brown rice for dinner could help them sleep better. Starchy carbohydrates in brown rice help to boost levels of the brain chemical serotonin, which regulates sleep. Brown rice also has a lower glycaemic index (GI) than white and so keeps blood-sugar levels steady for longer. This will help to prevent hunger from waking kids in the night, especially if they've eaten early in the evening. Plus brown rice is packed with magnesium, a good intake of which relaxes muscles and reduces stress, helping to prevent restless nights in teenagers who are worried about exams.

Beat constipation

Brown rice contains insoluble fibre and so can help to prevent constipation, a common problem in young children, often caused by poor fluid or fibre intakes. Insoluble fibre absorbs water, increasing the bulk and softness of the stools. This means they are easier to pass through the body, so your child won't need to strain when going to the toilet. Switching to brown rice means your child should also drink more fluids, though.

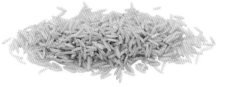
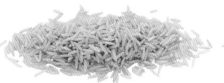
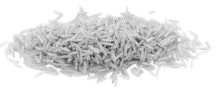

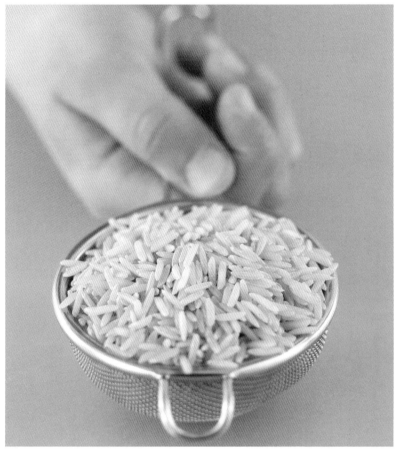

Ease asthma

Magnesium, which is in good supply in brown rice, may help to prevent or relieve the symptoms of asthma. Several studies have shown that asthma sufferers have low intakes of magnesium, a mineral that works its magic by relaxing the bronchial smooth muscle in the lungs, making breathing easier.

Release energy

Packing kids off to school with a salad made of brown rice could give them more energy in the afternoon. Brown rice contains manganese, a trace element, and vitamin B1, both of which help release energy from food.

Looking forward

Eating wholegrains such as brown rice has many long-term health benefits including lowering the risk of heart disease, cancer, obesity and diabetes (see Sweetcorn).

Won't eat...
Brown rice

Might eat...
Brown and white rice mixed together (cook separately then mix)

Will eat...
Chicken and vegetable stir-fried rice

Three ways
to get your kids to eat more brown rice

1 Mix brown rice into chilli, curry or stir-fries rather than serving it separately on the plate.

2 Add sweetcorn and peas to brown rice to add colour and texture.

3 Stuff peppers with brown rice and peas, cover in grated cheese and bake until the pepper softens and the cheese melts.

Why not try...

Fruity brown rice and vegetable salad (see page 124)
Nutritional facts per portion
194 kcal, 6.6 g fat (of which 1.1 g saturates), 8.9 g sugars, 0.1 g salt

Kedgeree (see page 124)
Nutritional facts per portion
180 kcal, 8.1 g fat (of which 1.8 g saturates), 5.4 g sugars, 0.2 g salt

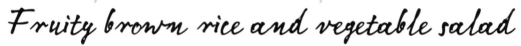

Fruity brown rice and vegetable salad

● Preparation time **15 mins** ● Cooking time **6–8 mins** ● Serves **4**

2 tbsp **olive oil**
2 **spring onions, finely chopped**
200 g (7 oz) **carrots, finely diced**
100 g (3½ oz) **celery, finely diced**
300 g (10 oz) **cooked brown rice**
100 g (3½ oz) **red and green seedless grapes, halved**
juice of ½ an orange
2 tbsp **mint, finely chopped**
pepper

1 Heat the oil in a large, nonstick frying pan or wok. Add the spring onions, carrots and celery, stir to mix and cook for 3–4 minutes or until the vegetables are just starting to soften.

2 Stir in the rice and mix well. Stir-fry for 3–4 minutes and then remove from the heat.

3 Stir in the grapes, orange juice and mint. Season with pepper and toss to mix well. Serve immediately or at room temperature.

Kedgeree

● Preparation time **30 mins** ● Cooking time **35–40 mins** ● Serves **6**

2 tbsp **olive oil**
1 **onion, finely chopped**
2 **garlic cloves, finely chopped**
1 tsp **fresh root ginger, finely grated**
2 tsp **cumin seeds**
2 tsp **mild curry powder**
1 tsp **ground cinnamon**
½ tsp **cardamom seeds, crushed**
1 **clove**
100 g (3½ oz) **dried split lentils, rinsed and drained**
200 g (7 oz) **brown basmati rice, rinsed and drained**
1 **carrot, cut into 1 cm (½ inch) dice**
100 g (3½ oz) **fine beans, cut into 1 cm (½ inch) pieces**
3 tbsp **fresh coriander leaves, finely chopped**
pepper
3 **hard-boiled eggs, quartered,**
200 g (7 oz) **natural low-fat yogurt**

1 Heat the oil in a large, heavy-based saucepan. Add the onion, garlic and ginger and stir-fry for 3–4 minutes. Stir in the cumin seeds, curry powder, cinnamon, cardamom and clove and stir-fry for a further minute.

2 Add the lentils, rice, carrot and beans and stir to mix well. Add 700 ml (25 fl oz) water and bring to the boil. Reduce the heat to low, cover and cook gently for about 30–40 minutes or until all the liquid is absorbed and the mixture is slightly sticky (do not be tempted to uncover the saucepan during this process). Remove from the heat and allow to stand, covered, for 10–12 minutes.

3 Fluff up the rice and lentil mixture with a fork and season with pepper. Stir in the coriander and spoon into a shallow serving dish. Garnish with the eggs and serve immediately with some whisked yogurt.

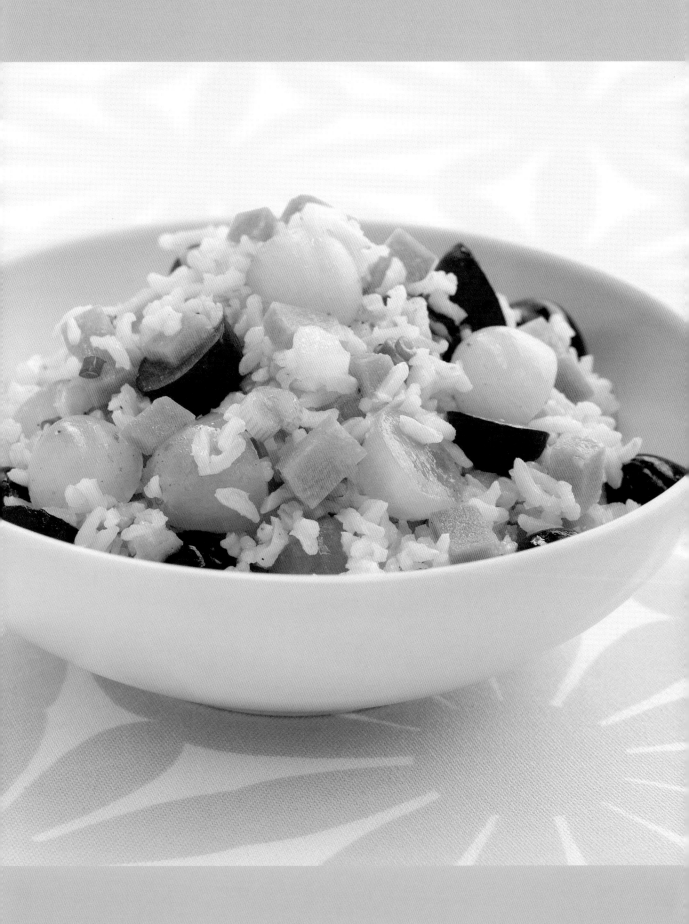

Index

Acknowledgements

Executive Editor: Nicola Hill

Editor: Emma Pattison

Executive Art Editor: Darren Southern

Designer: Maggie Town, One2Six Creative

Stylist: Sarah Waller

Senior Production Controller: Manjit Sihra

Picture Acknowledgements

Special Photography © Octopus Publishing Group Limited/Vanessa Davies.

Other photography:

Corbis UK Ltd. 102-104.

PhotoDisc 6 left, 6 right, 24 left, 24 right, 94-96, 98-100.